Biohacking,

Brain Health

And

Natural

Pain Management

How To Improve Your Life With Biohacks, How To Train
and Look After Your Brain and How To Manage Pain
Naturally

By Jim Russlan

circumstances is the author responsible for any losses, direct or indirect, which are incurred as a result of the use of information contained within this document, including, but not limited to, —errors, omissions, or inaccuracies.

Contents

Thank you for buying this book and I hope that you will find it useful. If you will want to share your thoughts on this book, you can do so by leaving a review on the Amazon page, it helps me out a lot.

Biohacking Guide

Learn How To Implement Biohacks into Your Daily Life
To Be Healthier, Feel Better and Achieve More

By Jim Russlan

Introduction to Biohacking Guide

Have you heard other individuals speaking about ideal Living and are questioning what it is and whether it could assist you to attain more of your objectives in life? In this book, we take a deeper look at what ideal living is everything about and how you can make modifications to your life to exploit its complete capacity.

Ideal living, at its heart, is everything about discovering the best balance in your life to assist you to attain the objectives that you have actually set yourself. It has to do with ending up being more efficient, more successful and creating more beneficial relationships in every part of your life. Working towards constant enhancement is at the core of ideal living.

Naturally, living ideally isn't something that constantly comes to us naturally. We need to incorporate modifications to enhance our physical and psychological wellness and we may do this by using particular life hacks.

What's a life hack? It's a basic modification that you can put in place that is going to transform how you do things. The point of a life hack is that it's a faster technique or way to increase your productivity and performance in all parts of your life.

Why are life hacks so advantageous for your physical and psychological wellness? The contemporary world is a frenzied and stressful location. We're all working harder than ever before, attempting to attain more in our private and working lives, while making every effort to remain healthy and fit both physically and psychologically at the same time.

It's a tall order. Streamlining how we live our lives can make a substantial distinction to how we deal with the world, and this is where life hacks can be important. These basic techniques are simple and fast to incorporate and can enhance and streamline how we live significantly. You'll discover that you'll quickly see favorable alterations that ripple out throughout all facets of your life.

Are you prepared to learn more about the life hacks that you can put in place in your own life? Then keep reading about 10 simple adjustments that are going to assist you in taking pleasure in the very best possible psychological and physical health every day of the year.

Chapter 1: Sleep Tracking

Sleep is a crucial aspect for both psychological and physical wellness. Without adequate sleep, you can't work efficiently daily. Not just does an absence of sleep affect your efficiency at work and home, it can, however, even induce you some severe medical problems. Poor quality sleep can cause psychological health issues like anxiety and depression, not to mention physical concerns like high blood pressure and cardiovascular disease, which can have enduring and serious consequences.

Nevertheless, while we understand that we ought to all be getting at least 8 hours of sleep every night, it could be hard to accomplish that objective. Whether you work shifts, have household obligations, or are having a hard time to get all your school or college work done, fitting in sufficient rest could be a severe obstacle. So, how can you fix that issue? The response might be tracking your sleep patterns.

Thanks to the most recent technology, you can have access to sleep tracking capability in the house. You can now purchase wearable sleep trackers that are going to track your sleep patterns to ensure that you can end up being more familiar with the length of time you sleep, the stages of sleep that you get to, and the quality of sleep.

Nowadays, we can tailor more things in our life than in the past. We can customize our clothing, phones, and houses, it makes sense to be able to individualize your sleep patterns too. Not everybody requires the exact same quantity of sleep every night, however, if you track your patterns, you can come to a greater understanding of the number of hours that is right for you.

If you're having sleep issues, a wearable sleep tracker is going to assist you in determining the reason behind your sleep concerns. At one time, the only choice was to go to a sleep laboratory to get an expert evaluation. Now, you can have comparable capability in your comfy bed. With the availability and precision of contemporary sleep trackers, you can find bothersome patterns and alter your routines for the better.

In case you track your sleep patterns, you are going to additionally start to wake at the optimum time. A lot of the most effective sleep trackers have a smart alarm to wake you when you're in the course of the lightest sleep phase. This prevents you from waking up dazed and irritable. Rather, you'll feel rested and prepared from the start for a more efficient day.

Sleep Tracking Benefits

If you buy a sleep tracker, you can enhance your sleep quality and, consequently, the lifestyle you can take pleasure in. More people are nervous and stressed than ever before, so getting adequate quality sleep is important.

If you are sleep deprived over prolonged durations, you are susceptible to medical issues, both physical and psychological. Cardiovascular disease, type II diabetes and breathing issues have actually all been related to sleeping disorders.

While we're really familiar with what we're doing throughout the day, throughout the night, our regimens frequently get forgotten. We're used to keeping track of habits throughout the day, from what we consume to just how much workout we get, so we ought to begin to do the identical thing throughout the nighttime hours.

If you track your sleep, the best advantage is that you'll begin to identify links in between your sleep patterns and total health. For instance, you'll find whether drinking coffee or consuming caffeine adversely affects your sleep or whether the alcohol that you consume impacts the quality of your rest.

You'll additionally discover whether the time at which you work out impacts your sleep patterns, whether working out at night or early morning is most advantageous for you, in addition to whether hanging out outdoors enhances or aggravates your rest. You'll have the ability to see if there is a link in between your utilization of computers and gadgets and the quality of your sleep, and just how much you sleep, or don't.

You'll even have the ability to figure out whether eating late at night or whether specific foods impact your sleep, and for ladies, whether their menstruation induces their sleep quality to change. By identifying these patterns, you can then quickly pick to embrace modifications in your way of life that are going to assist you to sleep better, along with additionally assisting you in being more efficient, more healthy and fit, and more effective in all parts of your life.

Chapter 2: Blue Light

More people are now ending up being more familiar with how blue light can impact our bodies, yet with increased gadget use, we're subjected to more of it than ever before. To delight in optimum wellness, we have to discover methods to lessen the quantity of blue light we permit ourselves to be subjected to. Why is this the case? Keep reading and find out more.

Blue Light's Impact on the Body?

Comprehending how light engages with our eyes is the trick to understanding why blue light is so negative for our wellness. Light is comprised of various colored waves, which all have their various energies. Red light is at the start of the apparent light spectrum. This has low energy waves and is less troublesome on the eyes, especially throughout the night. Blue light, nevertheless, has the greatest energy waves and this makes it harder for the eyes to process efficiently.

While high energy light waves are important for our everyday lives, it can prove to be hazardous if we are subjected to them at incorrect times. High energy light is obtained from the sun to manage sleep patterns efficiently. In the day, the light enters our eyes to discharge enzymes, bring our levels of melatonin down and assist us in awakening.

Melatonin manages our sleep cycles by means of biological rhythms. Nevertheless, this cycle is all too simple to interrupt. Extreme subjection to blue light can interrupt your body clock cycle. This is due to the fact that it minimizes the melatonin levels discharged by your body. If your body does not have sufficient melatonin at bedtime, you can't sleep effectively and you end up being tired.

Blue light is discharged by screens from laptops, tablets and smartphones and ultimately induces eye strain, near-sightedness and dry, itching eyes. Even worse, blue light impacts the retina and the cellular anchor and can induce advanced macular degeneration at an earlier age. Some professionals have actually even connected weight problems to melatonin disturbance in addition to the advancement of some types of cancer. Discovering methods to prevent extreme blue light exposure is, for that reason, important.

What to Do About Blue Light?

Some makers of gadgets are now acknowledging the damage that blue light can induce and are beginning to establish brand-new technological services to deal with the issue. Blue-filter covers are offered for buy for VR goggles, laptops and smartphones and some gadgets have actually now incorporated "night modes" into their model, which removes the blue light when you utilize your gadget at night hours to restrict your direct exposure.

Naturally, the apparent answer to the blue light direct exposure issue is merely to stay clear of utilizing any gadget throughout the night. Tablets and mobile phones ought to be kept out of the bedroom, and for numerous hours prior to bed, we ought to stay away from any gadget utilization. Sadly, this isn't constantly possible or perhaps desirable. So, how can we avoid the issue?

The solution could be to purchase a set of blue-light protective glasses. These are created with an HEV filter integrated. These enable you to utilize your gadgets whenever you like with no concern about direct exposure to blue light.

Blue light blocker glasses appear like a basic set of glasses, however, they have unique filters that stop high energy noticeable light from getting to the rear of the eye. They can either be bought as a standalone set of glasses or as a unique set of night-time glasses which could be used over a routine set of eyeglasses. In case you place these on your head around an hour prior to going to sleep, they are going to shut out all the blue light released from your gadgets and LED lights assisting you to improve sleep every night.

Chapter 3: Drink a Different Kind of Water

Another helpful hack that you can add to enhance your way of life is to consume alkaline water. This is among the current discoveries in the wellness and health sector, and it is one thing that can quickly be incorporated in your life.

All of us understand that water is essential to every tissue, cell and organ in our bodies. Nevertheless, a number of us stop working to remain as hydrated as we ought to by consuming adequate glasses of water. Now, brand-new research has actually revealed that we have to consume more water, however, the kind of water that we consume is similarly essential. Alkaline water is thought to be the very best thing for us to consume.

Why is Alkaline Water So Good?

Water is comprised of oxygen and hydrogen, with the variety of hydrogen ions in the water being determined as a pH figure.

Alkaline water consists of less hydrogen ions and has a greater pH level than basic faucet water. Water has a pH level which varies in between 0 and 14. 7 is stated to be neutral, with an equivalent balance in between acidic and alkaline. When the water has a pH level of beneath 7 it is acidic, and greater than 7 makes it alkaline. Water from the faucet in the United States normally has a pH of in between 4.3 and 5.3 depending upon where you live.

Those who proclaim the merits of alkaline water state that the bigger variety of hydrogen ions assists in offering more hydration when contrasted to routine water, especially if you have actually been exercising. They additionally think that routine faucet water that has an acidic pH triggers excessive acid to develop in your blood and cells leading to a series of health problems.

They think that alkaline water can minimize the quantity of acid in your bloodstream, offering your metabolic process an increase, boosting your energy levels, decreasing the aging procedure, enhancing your food digestion and even minimizing your bone loss. Some even state that it can starve cancer cells.

Alkaline water is an anti-oxidant that reduces the effects of the complimentary radicals which trigger cellular and DNA damage. Thanks to the tinier cluster size of the water, it can permeate the cells more quickly to hydrate you better, and its greater concentration of alkaline minerals such as magnesium, calcium and potassium assists to guarantee greater health.

Alkaline water is additionally abundant in oxygen which boosts the quantity of oxygen liquified in the blood, and thanks to its cleansing capabilities it can get rid of the accumulation of mucous on the walls of the colon to enhance your body's nutrient-absorbing capabilities.

This sort of water can eliminate the contaminants and acidic waste which has actually built up in your body while the adversely charged ions assist in increasing your awareness, psychological clearness, and energy levels. It can even assist in managing your weight and in remaining healthy because contaminants that are typically discovered in faucet water are eliminated.

How to Use Alkaline Water Properly

If you're all set to experience the advantages that drinking alkaline water can bring, you have to understand how you can acquire it. While you can purchase bottled alkaline water in shops, you can create it yourself with a water ionizer. A water ionizer is a compact system that links to the supply of water in your kitchen area. It performs low voltage electrolysis on your faucet water prior to consuming it or utilizing it in your kitchen for cooking or cleaning.

A water ionizer utilizes a specific accessory that reroutes the water from the faucet through a pipe into the system. In the system, water is filtered to remove the most typical contaminants which are discovered in routine faucet water. Next, the water which has actually been filtered hand down into a chamber which is geared up with titanium electrodes covered with platinum and it remains in this chamber where the electrolysis occurs.

Positive ions (or cations) converge at the negative electrodes. This develops decreased (or cathodic) water. On the other hand, the anions or negatively charged ions, converge at the positive electrode. This creates oxidized or anodic water.

The ionized water is guided to the tap while the oxidized water is guided to another pipe which leads to the sink. The ionized water can then be utilized for drinking or cooking. As a benefit, the oxidized water works as a disinfecting agent that could be utilized for cleaning up utensils, hands and food. If you purchase a water ionizer for your house, you can delight in all the advantages of alkaline water daily with no trouble.

Chapter 4: Red Light Treatment

RLT or Red Light Therapy is a restorative method which uses low-level red-light wavelengths to deal with a variety of skin issues like injuries, wrinkles and scars together with other conditions. How can it assist us in enhancing our total wellness? Keep reading.

What Is Red Light Therapy?

Throughout the 1990s, Red Light Therapy was utilized by researchers for cultivating plants in space and it was throughout this procedure that they found the extreme light generated by red LEDs (light-emitting diodes) promotes photosynthesis and development of the plant cells. It was then that red light started to be researched for its possible advantages in the realm of medication with tests being performed to see if RLT boosted the energy in human cells to deal with bone density issues, sluggish recovery of injuries and muscle atrophy.

There are numerous sorts of RLT with both beauty and medical applications. It can deal with severe conditions like slow-to-heal injuries and psoriasis, along with cosmetic concerns such as stretch marks and wrinkles.

Red Light Therapy functions by generating biochemical results in the cells to enhance their mitochondria. These are the cell's powerhouse where the energy of the cell is produced. ATP is the energy-carrying particle that could be discovered within the cells and when RLT boosts the mitochondria's function, it creates more ATP. Consequently, cells have more energy which allows them to revitalize themselves, fix damage and function better.

Unlike other IPL or laser treatments, RLT does not harm the surface area of the skin. Rather, it promotes skin regrowth to use a host of advantages consisting of:

- Promotion of injury recovery and tissue repair.

- Treatment of carpal tunnel syndrome

- Enhanced hair growth

- Decrease of psoriasis sores

- Stimulated recovery of injuries that are sluggish to recover

- Decrease of adverse effects from cancer treatments

- Relief of discomfort and tightness in those experiencing rheumatoid arthritis

- Enhanced skin tone and boosted collagen for decreased wrinkles

- Fixing of sun damage

- Enhanced joint health in people with osteoarthritis

- Prevention of repeating fever blisters

- Relief of discomfort and swelling

- Reduced scars

As you can see, there are a number of reasons why you ought to think about having Red Light Treatment to enhance your total health and wellness.

How to Take Advantage Of Red Light Treatment

You can discover red light treatment in use for cosmetic functions in spas, tanning salons and gyms. Nevertheless, there are additionally a number of FDA-approved RLT gadgets that you can purchase for usage in your home. While these will not be as effective as those which you can discover in medical usage, they work at combating undesirable indications of early aging like fine lines, age spots and wrinkles. If you wish to deal with a medical condition, nevertheless, you'll have to talk about the alternatives offered to you with a physician to guarantee you enjoy optimum advantages.

RLT is pain-free and secure if the gadgets are utilized correctly. There have actually been stories of some individuals getting burns due to gadget rust, damaged wires or due to the fact that they dropped off to sleep with their system still in place. Nevertheless, when the guidelines are followed effectively, red light treatment isn't hazardous. It is, nevertheless, really essential to utilize eye safety because red light can harm the eyes.

Considering that RLT has actually been demonstrated to have appealing outcomes when it concerns dealing with a number of skin issues, it's well worth including red light treatment into your routine skincare program. If you're worried about your signs, you might want to consult your medical professional initially to make certain that RLT is the very best choice for you, but for lots of people, the advantages of red light treatment make the investment in a red light-emitting gadget well worth it.

Chapter 5: Be More Active

All of us understand that we ought to get lots of exercises to remain in peak physical and psychological shape. Nevertheless, despite this prevalent understanding, a lot of us still aren't getting the advised quantity of activity on an everyday or weekly basis. The next crucial hack to include into your life is to include more workout every day. How can you accomplish this when you're on a tight schedule? Here, we take a look at a few of the advantages of being more physical and some innovative methods to fir more activity into your daily life.

The Issues of an Inactive Way of life

You'll most likely have heard in the media that a lot of people are living an inactive way of life, however, what does this imply?

Inactive living is living where you do not do enough exercise frequently. The present suggestions by the CDC are that we all ought to do a minimum of 150 minutes of moderate exercise daily or, additionally, 75 minutes of energetic workout. Walking 10,000 steps daily is suggested to enhance your health and to minimize the possible health threats which happen due to lack of exercise.

The WHO states that as much as 85 percent of the world's population isn't sufficiently physically active and this makes the inactive way of life the 4th leading threat around the world. Typically, we are led to believe that eating healthily and taking some aerobic workout can balance out all the impacts triggered by too much time taking a seat. Nevertheless, proof now reveals that if you work out for half an hour a day, you still might not be able to reduce the possible damage. The very best option seems to lower the quantity of time taking a seat and increase the quantity of time we devote to moving daily.

The inactive way of life leads to many unfavorable impacts. Whether you're working at a desk or driving a bus or taxi, you are placing yourself at the danger of the following issues:

- A greater danger of establishing specific cancers

- A greater possibility of struggling with specific cardiovascular issues

- A higher likelihood of establishing anxiety and depression

- A higher likelihood of ending up being overweight or obese

- Greater high blood pressure

- Lowered skeletal muscle mass

- Raised cholesterol levels

It has actually been approximated that, worldwide, inactive way of life induces 7 percent of all cases of coronary cardiovascular disease, 6 percent of all instances of type II diabetes, 11 percent of all instances of breast cancer, and 11 percent of all instances of colon cancer. It has actually even been disclosed that a sedentary way of life leads to more deaths every year than cigarette smoking.

We are more inactive today than we ever have actually been before since innovation has actually altered how we live our lives. 50 years back, less individuals utilized vehicles and had desk jobs. They additionally had more physical leisure activities and hobbies instead of viewing Television and playing computer games. The amount of inactive tasks has actually grew by over 80 percent since the 50s, and when we include into that the reality that we now have longer typical working weeks, that is a lot more time devoted to being in a seated position.

It's obvious that discovering methods to neutralize the unfavorable effect of the inactive way of life is important, however, fortunately, there are numerous biohacking modifications to enhance your health, wellness and fitness in general.

How To Be More Active

All of us understand that maintaining our physical health ought to be a leading concern, however, we're likewise busier than ever before in our lives. With duties like looking after senior parents or kids, a busy social life and demanding jobs, we're all under pressure in a frenzied speed of life. Naturally, the most apparent method of getting more active is to go to a gym or to reserve an hour every early morning or night to exercise in the house. Nevertheless, this simply isn't feasible for some individuals.

Lots of people are frightened by the concept of heading to the gym, while discovering the time to fit physical activity into a day-to-day routine can be practically inconceivable. For that reason, discovering methods to end up being more active while setting about our routine activities is the very best option.

Here are a couple of easy hacks to change your day-to-day regimen into a much healthier one:

- Change to a standing desk instead of a routine one. Office workers feel connected to their desks for much of the day, however, if you make the easy modification to standing instead of sitting, you'll discover that you're less stiff and slow when your day comes to a conclusion. Standing utilizes a lot more muscles when contrasted to sitting, and proof has actually revealed that standing every thirty minutes and walking around can minimize your odds of passing away early. Even better, it promotes much better posture which, in turn, lowers tension and exhaustion while urging much better performance and steadier breathing. If you wish to take things a step further, why not change to a treadmill desk rather. This is going to assist you to remain a lot more active while you work, and you can jog or walk during your important work activities.

- Take the stairs instead of the elevator. Walking up a slope is much better for you than strolling on a flat surface area, so select the stairs for optimum benefit when becoming active. Research reveals that if you climb up the stairs simply 3 times weekly, your cardiorespiratory physical fitness is going to enhance. Your leg muscles are going to end up being more powerful, and you'll additionally burn more calories for simpler bodyweight upkeep.

- Include basic workouts into your regimen. If you do not have adequate hours in the day to reach the gym, include some muscle exercises into your everyday program rather. Doing squats while at your desk or dips on your workplace chair will not take much work and it can assist you in enhancing your general physical fitness and health. You can even include small changes like stabilizing on one leg while brushing your teeth or doing customized push-ups versus your counter top.

- Ditch the vehicle. Rather than driving to work or the shop, attempt cycling or strolling rather. You'll discover that it is going to bring you physical and psychological advantages.

- Utilize a resistance ball rather than a routine chair. Whether you're at work or in your home, changing your standing chair for a resistance ball is going to assist to immediately align your spinal column, enhance your posture and motivate you to stretch and move more frequently. You can even do some little workouts simultaneously like modified sit-ups to involve core muscle strength.

- Take brief strolls throughout the day. Throughout your lunch break, rather than vegetating at your desk, take a fast walk around the block rather. Simply a ten-minute walk daily can offer you favorable physical and psychological advantages. An exercise does not have to take an hour. Simply 10 or 15 minutes of physical activity provides advantages too and is going to get your heart pumping while additionally assisting you to enhance your psychological health.

Chapter 6: Mindfulness

The contemporary world is definitely a busy one. Hurrying to perform all you have to do could be really difficult, so it's no surprise that more people discover that we have actually lost our connection with the present moment. A number of us discover that we're losing out on the satisfaction of the minute. We neglect how we're feeling at any time and this can cause unfavorable repercussions physically and psychologically in our lives.

Did you get up feeling rested today? Did you observe those flowers flowering in your street today? Did you hear the birds singing as you got to work? If the response to those was no, you ought to consider practicing mindfulness.

What Is Mindfulness?

The term "mindfulness" is utilized to explain the practice of focusing all your attention intentionally on the minute you remain in and accepting your feelings and sensations with no judgement. It has actually been shown to be a significant part in attaining general joy and decreasing tension levels.

Mindfulness has its origins in Buddhism, Nevertheless, practically every religion includes some kind of prayer or meditation method to move your thought patterns far from typical fixations and towards gratitude of the present moment.

Practicing mindfulness has actually been demonstrated to bring a wealth of enhancements to both physical and mental signs, assisting in bringing favorable change to mindsets, habits and health. When you're conscious, you can take pleasure in life's moments when they happen. This enables you to engage more completely with activities and assist you in coping better with unfavorable occasions in your life.

If you concentrate on the now, you'll have a minimized likelihood of getting caught up with your concerns about things you have actually carried out in your past or things you'll carry out in the future. You'll have less fixations with success and self-confidence while additionally having the ability to form deeper and better connections with other individuals.

Mindfulness has actually been demonstrated to enhance your physical health. It can assist in enhancing heart health, eliminating tension, lowering your high blood pressure, lowering discomfort, enhancing your sleep and even reducing intestinal issues. On the other hand, it provides a host of psychological health advantages consisting of the relief of substance abuse, depression, anxiety, eating disorders and OCD.

How Does It Work?

Specialists think that, partially, mindfulness works by assisting in allowing individuals to accept feelings and experiences rather than responding with hostility or avoidance.

Mindfulness could be practiced in lots of ways., Nevertheless, the main objective of mindfulness methods is to end up being more alert and concentrated and unwinded by paying very close attention intentionally to the ideas and feelings you experience at any given minute without judgement. Consequently, your mind can refocus efficiently on today.

There are numerous mindfulness methods. Nevertheless, this is a standard guide to including mindfulness practices into your life:

- Start by taking a seat silently and concentrating on your breathing patterns. Additionally, you can concentrate on a word or mantra which you restate to yourself quietly. Allow your ideas to go without judgement, returning to concentrating on your mantra or breathing.

- Note the subtle experiences in your body like itching or tingling. Once again, do not evaluate them, simply enable them to pass. Concentrate your focus on each part of the body from your head to your toes.

- Note the noises, tastes, sights, smells and touches around you. Once again, without judgement, simply permit them to come and go.

- Handle your cravings, whether they are for a pattern of habits or for a compound. Acknowledge the sensations, however, permit them to go through you without judgement.

You can start practicing mindfulness alone by utilizing tai chi, yoga or other meditation techniques. You merely have to develop concentration, observe the sensations and ideas streaming through your body without judgement, and see the experiences that you experience. With time and practice, you'll discover that you end up being more pleased and more self-aware.

Tips for Introducing Mindfulness Practice into Your Life

If you're prepared to present mindfulness practice into your life, you might begin participating in a class or purchase a meditation CD to start practicing. There are, nevertheless, less conventional methods you can embrace. Here are some leading ideas to assist in breaking the ice to mindfulness:

- Select an activity throughout which you'll engage in mindfulness. It might be when you're walking, eating or showering.

- Begin by concentrating on the feelings your body is experiencing.

- Breathe gradually through the nose. Permit the air to move downwards to your lower stomach and permit your stomach to totally broaden.

- Breathe gradually out through the mouth.

- Consider the feelings you experience whenever you breathe out or breathe in.

- Gradually, proceed with your activity with consideration.

- Totally engage all your senses. Consider every touch, sight and noise. Relish each experience.

- If you understand your mind is straying from the present activity, bring your focus back carefully onto the sensations you're experiencing.

You can't hurry mindfulness. Nevertheless, the more frequently you practice, the more you'll discover that it works. Be ready for the truth that it'll typically take about 20 minutes up until your mind begins to settle. Practicing the above strategies for brief durations a couple of times a week is the very best method to begin, then you can muster up to longer durations of meditation on more days of the week.

Chapter 7: Whole Foods

Although all of us understand that we ought to consume more whole foods, it could be all too appealing to draw on the processed food that we discover in restaurants and shops all over. Fast food is an ever-present feature of life on the planet today.

The existence of McDonald's, KFC and Burger King in shopping centers all over the nation is just motivating more people to snack on that from an early age. More individuals today are consuming processed food than ever in the past, however, the trade-off for ease is a host of health problems for both the mind and body.

Why is unhealthy food such an issue, and how could it have an unfavorable influence on your wellness? Here, we take a closer look at why entire foods are a much better option in your everyday diet plan and how you can present them better into your life.

The Unhealthy Food Issue

The definition of unhealthy food is food which is inadequate in nutrients and thick in calories. Over the past couple of years, comfort and junk food intake have actually significantly increased, and today, approximately a quarter of the population primarily takes in processed foods. Consequently, there has actually been an increasing epidemic of persistent illness.

The primary issue connected with the intake of unhealthy food routinely are weight problems. It is anticipated that the weight problem rate in 2050 in the U.S.A. alone with reach 42 percent. Kids taking in processed food frequently consume more carbs, fats, and processed sugars and less fiber than they require. Consuming 187 extra calories daily than they need, it's not surprising that 6 pounds of weight is put on each year, increasing their odds of establishing heart disease and diabetes, to name a few persistent illnesses.

Another issue developing from processed food usage is the danger of establishing diabetes. Insulin levels increase whenever you take in processed sugars which are discovered in white flour, sodas and other food which does not have the important nutrients and fiber to metabolize carbs successfully. If you consume unhealthy food throughout the day, your insulin levels can end up being chronically high leading to insulin resistance gradually. This triggers type II diabetes to arrive.

If you get rid of fiber, vitamins and minerals from your eating plan, you can end up being nutritionally lacking. This can lead to low energy levels, sleep disruptions, low performance, and state of mind swings. High levels of salt discovered in processed food additionally lead to the overconsumption of salt. This leads to heart, liver and kidney illness along with high blood pressure.

Not all the issues arising from the usage of unhealthy food are physical. Some are psychological too. A 2015 research study demonstrated that individuals on high glycemic eating plans suffered more from depression than those who had a low GI eating plan. Because junk food-heavy eating plans are so bad for us, it stands to reason that we ought to try to find a much better eating plan that promotes health and well- being. This is where whole foods can enter into play.

What Are Whole Foods?

This term is utilized to describe food which is nearest to its natural state. They benefit us since they carry more nutrients than packaged and processed foods. Professionals recommend that we ought to all be going for whole foods comprising around 75 percent of our everyday eating plan. This is going to assist us to remain healthy, without illness, with slower aging.

What foods should we be consuming?

Whole foods consist of fruits and veggies which have not been processed along with whole grains like millet, oats, quinoa, buckwheat, cornmeal, rye, and wild rice. We ought to additionally be consuming more beans and beans like lentils and chickpeas along with more nuts and seeds. Wholefoods additionally consist of those stemmed from animal origins consisting of eggs, fish, poultry, seafood and lean red meat like veal, pork, beef and lamb.

If you consume unprocessed foods, you'll have the ability to take in the optimum quantity of day-to-day nutrients you need for total wellness and health, and in the very best possible percentages.

Wholefoods consist of various nutrients all in a single food consisting of vitamins, minerals, fiber, vital fats, and phytonutrients. They are additionally really abundant in substances which can't be manufactured in the body and which, for that reason, have to be acquired by means of your eating plan. For instance, valine, an amino acid, can not be made by the body itself, and for that reason, needs to be provided by means of what you consume. It is important for tissue repair work and muscle metabolic processes, so incorporating lots of whole foods in your everyday routine is necessary.

When you consume entire foods in their natural state, you can take advantage of the synergy result of the nutrients in the food interacting to benefit your body's healthy performance. For instance, tryptophan, an amino acid, needs B vitamins to become serotonin. Additionally, entire foods are abundant in the anti-oxidants which reduce the effects of free radicals and battle issues like cancer and cardiovascular disease.

One More Reason to Eat Whole Foods

For several years, specialists have actually been informing us that fruits and veggies are important for our wellness. Nevertheless, a lot of us still discover it hard to incorporate enough of them into our eating plans. Yet, entire foods can stop us from ending up being ill and assist in preventing the issue of weight problems.

Lots of research studies have actually uncovered that consuming more whole foods is going to provide your body with important nutrition sources consisting of calcium, fiber, magnesium, B vitamins, protein, Vitamin D, potassium and necessary fats which guarantee your body's cells work in the proper way. Foods that are processed are challenging to absorb correctly and can make you feel tired and sick.

When you include more entire foods into your life, you'll experience a host of advantages consisting of:

- Enhanced blood glucose levels. Processed foods consist of insulin growth factor that makes your blood glucose levels greater. As a result, you experience blood glucose swings and yearnings. Entire foods will not create these spikes and are going to assist you to keep balance throughout the day.

- Enhanced food digestion. Entire foods consist of great deals of fiber, which is a crucial nutrient for food digestion. This fiber is natural and is going to assist you to feel fuller for longer while additionally supporting your food digestion and reducing your blood glucose levels as it breaks down gradually in the body.

- Greater energy levels-- the body is more competent of obtaining energy from healthy foods than processed ones, so you'll begin to feel more invigorated with a quicker metabolic process when you consume more entire foods.

- Minimized discomfort-- processed foods have high inflammatory properties. Given that they are acidic in nature, they develop pH level imbalances which can lead to persistent pain condition signs worsening. Entire foods keep your body more alkaline, and for that reason, devoid of swelling and discomfort.

How to Consume More Whole Foods

Do you like the advantages of consuming more entire foods, however, do not understand how to include them to your eating plan? Here are a couple of fast ideas to point you in the appropriate direction:

- Change to conventional oats instead of instant oat cereals. Instant oats are going to typically have oat bran disposed of. This implies that a great deal of the vitamins and fiber have actually been disposed of, lowering its dietary worth.

- Change to whole fruit and veggies instead of packaged juice. When fruit is juiced, it ends up being a focused sugar source, and this raises your blood glucose level far more quickly when compared to entire fruits. Juicers additionally dispose of the pulp and skin of the fruit, so flavonoids and anti-oxidants are removed. Packaged juices additionally have additional sugar combined with chemicals and preservatives.

- Change to fresh fish instead of canned or frozen fish. Fish consist of vital fats that are typically disposed of or minimized throughout the product packaging procedure. You require omega 3 fats to keep your nervous, immune, cardiovascular and reproductive systems working correctly.

You can quickly discover entire foods for sale in supermarket if you go shopping in the aisles committed to fresh food. As you move towards the center of the shop, bear in mind that you'll discover more processed foods, so attempt to go shopping on the external edges of the shop. You'll additionally discover entire foods in farmers' markets and at natural food shops.

You do not have to entirely eradicate all processed food from your life to remain healthy, however, if you can boost your wholefood usage to around 75 percent, you'll take pleasure in much greater health and overall wellness.

Chapter 8: Probiotics

The majority of us tend to believe that germs are bad and harmful for us., Nevertheless, this isn't the case. There are numerous kinds of germs that are helpful for our bodies. These live micro-organisms are referred to as probiotics, or friendly germs, and can assist in making your body much healthier.

There are various kinds of probiotics that deliver various advantages for your wellness and health. They operate in the GI system to reinforce the immune system, stopping unsafe germs from ending up being connected to the interior wall of the intestinal tracts while enhancing the balance and function of the intestinal lining's natural microflora.

Typically, the human body has an ideal balance of bacteria, nevertheless, there are particular medical elements which can lead to imbalances.

Consequently, the disease-causing germ numbers can grow greatly. Unneeded use of antibiotics, intestinal issues, surgical treatment, taking PPIs, persistent stress, sensitivity to gluten, and even the typical American diet can trigger such imbalances.

Fortunately, there are methods to remedy the balance of bacteria for much better general wellness and health. The very best method is to add probiotics to your day-to-day eating plan.

What Are Probiotics?

Probiotic is a term utilized to illustrate the live germs which exist in yogurt and fermented foods. They can benefit your digestion system by delivering the balance of the friendly and bad germs in your microbiome in alignment. This guarantees you have a lower threat of experiencing various medical illnesses and conditions.

Probiotics could be made from health food sources like yogurt and kefir, however, they can likewise be made from foods which have actually been improved with probiotics along with from professional supplements. It's typically ideal to get your probiotics from healthy food sources, nevertheless.

Probiotics take numerous shapes and can be discovered in these foods:

- Sauerkraut and unpasteurized kimchi.

- Miso soup

- Soft cheese and enriched milk.

- Sour pickles in saltwater

- Sourdough bread

Here are a few of the most helpful probiotic foods that you can take pleasure in every day:

- Yogurt-- this is a leading probiotic source because it consists of milk which has actually been fermented by friendly germs like bifidobacterial and lactic acid germs. Not just can yogurt increase your bone health, it can minimize hypertension and eliminate undesirable signs related to IBS (irritable bowel syndrome). Not every kind of yogurt includes probiotics, so you have to just select yogurts with active or live cultures.

- Kefir-- this probiotic fermented milk beverage is created from cow or goat milk with included kefir grains. Once again, kefir can reinforce the bones, aid with gastrointestinal problems, and shield the body from infections.

- Sauerkraut-- this is created from shredded cabbage which has actually been fermented with lactic acid germs. Not just is sauerkraut loaded with vitamins and fiber; it additionally includes manganese, salt and iron in addition to anti-oxidants which enhance eye health. You have to make certain that the sauerkraut you have actually picked is unpasteurized to experience its probiotic advantages.

- Tempeh-- this item is created from fermented soybeans and is prominent as a replacement for meat. The fermentation procedure implies that you can take in more minerals from tempeh. It is additionally an abundant source of vitamin B12 while additionally having probiotic advantages.

- Kimchi-- this spicy, fermented Korean meal is normally created from cabbage which has actually been seasoned with chili pepper, garlic, ginger, scallions and salt. It additionally includes Lactobacillus kimchi which benefits your gastrointestinal health.

- Miso-- this Japanese flavoring is created from fermented soybeans. Typically made into soup, miso is an exceptional source of protein and fiber and is loaded with plant substances, vitamins and minerals

- Kombucha-- this fermented black or green tea drink is from Asia.

- Pickles-- gherkins are fermented in salt and are an outstanding source of probiotic germs which enhance gastrointestinal health.

- Buttermilk-- standard buttermilk is the liquid that is left after creating butter. It consists of probiotics in addition to important vitamins and minerals.

- Natto-- this fermented soybean item resembles tempeh and miso which consists of Bacillus subtilis. It is additionally high in protein and vitamin K2.

- Some cheeses-- although lots of cheeses are fermented, they do not all consist of probiotics. Just those that have active and live cultures do. Cottage cheese, cheddar, gouda and mozzarella are all fine examples of cheeses in which the friendly germs make it through the procedure of aging.

There are numerous probiotic foods which you can include in your eating plan, nevertheless, if you do not like all of them, you might constantly attempt a probiotic supplement which could be taken daily to enhance your total wellness and health.

Chapter 9: Cryotherapy

Although cryotherapy has actually been around for a long time, it has only just recently reached widespread attention. This is due to the fact that celebs have actually begun to proclaim its virtues, specifically sports stars who state that it assists in improving their healing time after exercise.

Cryotherapy has actually been growing as a fad in spas and health centers because of its appeal with celebs and professional athletes. Those who have this treatment take pleasure in quicker healing times after exercising and think that the sub-zero temperature levels can diminish asthma, anxiety and stress and arthritis, in addition to making the skin look younger.

Cryotherapy sessions can take a number of shapes. The most common include standing in a whole-body cryo-chamber. This chamber is a can-like enclosure with an open-top, so the user's head constantly stays out. On the other hand, the remainder of the body is subjected to sub-zero temperature levels.

When having WBC, you use gloves, underclothing and socks to avoid your extremities establishing frostbite. Each session just lasts a number of minutes and although it might feel a little uneasy and odd, it isn't undesirable or uncomfortable. There are additionally targeted cryotherapy treatments that include just exposing one part of the body to sub-zero temperature levels. This works for easing discomfort in a particular location.

The concept behind cryotherapy is to decrease the body temperature level to such a degree that the "fight or flight" mode is launched. This triggers the body to deliver the blood from the extremities to the heart where it is quickly oxygenated and pumped filled with nutrients. On departing the chamber, the newly oxygenated blood is pumped outwards back around the body once again to enhance healing and recovery.

What is Good About Cryotherapy?

Cryotherapy is thought to provide a host of psychological and physical advantages. These consist of:

- Decrease of migraine signs-- cryotherapy is thought to deal with migraines because it numbs and cools the nerves around the neck, cooling off the blood which goes through the intracranial vessels.

- Minimized nerve inflammation-- cryotherapy is utilized by professional athletes to numb discomfort from inflamed nerves. It works in dealing with neuromas, severe injuries, pinched nerves or persistent pain.

- Manages mood disorders-- when the entire body undergoes sub-zero temperature levels there is a physiological hormone reaction in the body that includes the release of noradrenaline, adrenaline and endorphins. This can assist those who experience anxiety and depression to experience a much better state of mind.

- Lowered arthritic discomfort-- individuals struggling with arthritis can experience less discomfort when having either whole body or localized cryotherapy.

- It deals with skin issues-- if you experience skin problems like atopic dermatitis, you might discover that cryotherapy can assist in alleviating itching and dryness. Cryotherapy lowers swelling while additionally enhancing the levels of anti-oxidants in the blood which assists in enhancing the condition of the skin. For the identical reason, it's additionally useful in alleviating cases of acne.

- Enhanced weight reduction-- weight gain is a significant issue worldwide today; nevertheless, cryotherapy has actually been discovered to have some weight-loss advantages considering that it accelerates the metabolic process for numerous hours following treatment. This suggests that those who have WBC can successfully burn more calories after having a treatment session.

These are simply a few of the advantages that have actually been reported after having cryotherapy. As you can see, there are numerous reasons you may wish to think about trying it out on your own to see what benefits it can bring you for your wellness and health.

Chapter 10: Cleanse Your Air

Are you concerned about impurities in the air? Do you struggle with asthma or allergies? Do you have animals in your house, or do you reside with a cigarette smoker? If the response to any of these is yes, you ought to think about taking a look at methods to cleanse your air. Here, we take a better look at a few of the reasons that more individuals are selecting to buy an air purifier as a leading hack for a much healthier way of life.

Why Should I Cleanse my Air?

We frequently think that the air within our houses is healthy and clean to breathe. Nevertheless, it might come as a surprise to discover that it could be just as infected and contaminated as the air outdoors.

Smells, dust, animal dander, mold and smoke are simply a few of the pollutants that you can discover in the air within your house and there are some toxins within your house which exist in quantities 5 times higher than in the air outdoors. It's no surprise, then, that many individuals experience asthma and allergies. Discovering a method to catch undesirable particles from the air like dust and pollen is important.

So, how to determine if the air in your house requires cleansing? Here are simply a few of the reasons to think about:

- You have animals. If you have a cat or dog , you might wind up experiencing breathing issues. They shed dander onto surface areas of your house which can not be gotten rid of by vacuuming alone. Cleansing the air is the very best method to be certain of eliminating this issue successfully.

- You experience hay fever, allergic reactions or asthma. Throughout the summertime and spring, hay fever is a typical issue due to the pollen particles which are in the air. These aggravate the eyes and can trigger asthma. Cleansing the air is going to get rid of these irritants so you can stay comfy all season long.

- You have a mold issue in your home. If your house is damp or vulnerable to damp, you might discover that mold is an issue. Restrooms and kitchen areas are problematic zones and without eliminating the spores from the air, you might establish breathing issues. Cleansing the air removes this possibility.

- You have dust mites. Dust mites remain in everybody's house and can trigger allergies on the skin in addition to breathing issues. If you cleanse the air, you will not need to stress over this issue.

- You reside with a cigarette smoker. Smoke from cigarettes can dangle in the air for a very long time triggering breathing issues in vulnerable people, not to mention undesirable smells. If you cleanse the air, this will not be a problem.

- You do not like cooking smells. Whether you live close to next-door neighbors who prepare strong-smelling foods or whether you prepare them yourself, you do not want the smells remaining around your house. An air purifier can get rid of the undesirable smells.

- You have jeopardized immunity. Airborne infection particles can move in between people when they sneeze or cough. If you cleanse the air inside your house, your entire household is going to have much better health and general wellness.

- You have an infant. Young kids are specifically at risk of air-borne bacteria and viruses. They might additionally be more at risk when they're exposed to hazardous pollutants and contaminants in the indoor environment.

Cleansing the air is going to offer your kids the very best likelihood of taking pleasure in ideal health.

- You live near to a roadway or a farm. If you reside in a location which is at high danger of contamination, you ought to cleanse the air inside your house to keep the threat of contamination to a minimum.

As you can see, there are numerous reasons for thinking about cleansing the air in your house to enhance your total wellness and health.

How Can I Keep the Air in my House Pure?

There are a number of things you may do to keep the air in your house pure and tidy. Among the very best is to buy an air purifier. This is a gadget that has numerous filters in addition to a fan to absorb the air and distribute it while catching the contaminants and particles and pressing tidy air back to the home.

When selecting an air purifier, you ought to ensure to select one which has a HEPA filter (high-efficiency particle air filter). These capture particles of a series of sizes in an extremely fine multi-layered web created from fiberglass threads. This airtight filter guarantees that even the smallest ultra-fine particles are caught so they can not be launched into the environment to trigger issues. You ought to pick an air purifier that is big enough to successfully clean up the air in the area which you reside in, and which has a tidy air shipment rate of over 350. This is going to make sure that the air stays as pure and clean as possible.

There are additionally some other things you may do to enhance the quality of the air inside your house. For a start, although it might sound counter-intuitive, you can keep the windows open, producing a cross-draft whenever feasible by opening the window on opposite sides of your spaces. This is going to guarantee that undesirable contaminants and pollutants will not end up being caught inside your home, triggering your health issue.

You ought to additionally vacuum your floors regularly to eliminate dust mites which can trigger skin and breathing issues, and utilize exhaust fans in your laundry locations, restroom and kitchen area to prevent mold from developing and triggering breathing troubles and major diseases.

You ought to stay clear of lighting a wood fire inside your house and prevent cigarette smoking within your home as this is going to assist in enhancing the quality of air inside your house too. Smoke can trigger breathing issues while secondary smoke from tobacco can be really damaging to your health, even triggering cancer sometimes.

Obviously, you ought to additionally keep in mind to frequently alter the filters in your air purifier, vacuum and ventilation system to make sure that the air inside your home remains clean and healthy. A blocked filter can not easily catch particles and pollutants, so you have to make certain to remain on top of the altering schedule to make sure that maximum contaminants are gotten rid of from the air that you and your household breathe daily.

Conclusion of Biohacking Guide

We are residing in an extremely stressed contemporary world and more people than ever before are living a frenzied way of life. Consequently, we experience a host of psychological, physical and emotional health problems varying from allergic reactions and asthma to depression and anxiety. It's not surprising that, then, that a lot of individuals are trying to find methods to enhance their wellness to ensure that they can stay clear of the tension that today's lifestyle can bring.

While there is lots of guidance out there about various methods to decrease the issues connected with contemporary living, a few of the choices recommended could be hard to put in place and could be way too much of a hassle. That's why easy and fast biohacks exist. The biohacks that are recommended here represent a few of the most effective methods to offer your life an overhaul for the better. By carrying out a couple of easy and little modifications in various locations of your life, you can take pleasure in much better wellness.

Possibly you're experiencing a particular health issue such as anxiety, asthma or a skin problem. Or maybe you're simply searching for a much better means to live without putting yourself at risk of health issue establishing. In either case, there is sure to be a minimum of one biohack here that is going to change the manner in which you handle your daily affairs.

You can purchase easy tools for your house that are going to restrict your direct exposure to blue light, eliminate contaminants and pollutants from the air or provide your water an alkaline pH. It's extremely simple to put such modifications in place and the advantages that you'll experience are certainly considerable.

Additionally, why not attempt one of the treatments that were recommended such as Cryotherapy or Red Light Therapy. Both are simple and fast and can bring you a host of health advantages that can assist you in getting even more pleasure out of your life.

Even if you're on a tight spending plan and can't pay for the cost of heading to a wellness spa for cryotherapy treatments or acquiring a water ionizer for your home water system, there are still biohack modifications that you can implement that are entirely free of charge and which can still bring you a wealth of psychological and physical advantages. By just including mindfulness and meditation into your day-to-day program, you can give yourself

more defense from psychological health issue, while adding probiotic foods such as yogurt or sauerkraut into your eating plan can significantly enhance your food digestion and assist you to attain higher health in numerous parts of your life.

Getting more active is another outstanding biohack that costs you absolutely nothing. By merely getting up and strolling more throughout your working day, picking to walk instead of driving or taking the bus and utilizing the stairs instead of the elevator, you can increase your general physical fitness level, assist yourself in preserving a healthy body weight and even provide your psychological health a much-needed enhancement.

Although it might sound difficult to alter your life for the better, you can see from these 10 easy biohacks that it doesn't need to be hard to turn your life around for the better. Begin by making one modification, and after that, in time, you can begin to make more modifications up until you have actually lastly attained ideal welness and health. When you feel wonderful daily, you'll be happy that you began biohacking your life!

Brain Health 101

Beginner's Guide to Habits, Strategies and Diet for Training Your Brain So You Can Get The Most Out of It to Be Smarter, More Focused, More Alert and More Creative

By Jim Russlan

Introduction to Brain Health 101

A great deal of individuals have an interest in fitness and health nowadays and to that end, they are going to devote a great deal of time in the gym or out running in a bid to attempt and put on more muscle and increase their physical conditioning.

However, while this is an exceptional objective, it's possibly an example of us having the incorrect goals. Why? Since nowadays, we do not utilize our bodies half as much as we utilize our brains. Our brains are what we utilize for most of the professions nowadays, they are what we utilize to handle our relationships and they are what we utilize to manage cash, learn and more.

So if you will devote time exercising your body, it just stands to reason that you ought to devote a minimum of the identical quantity of time exercising your brain.

So why aren't more individuals currently training their brains? Mostly, this boils down to the truth that many individuals do not understand rather the degree to which their brains could be trained, or rather the degree to which their brain function could be enhanced through merely following the most effective health practices-- through the appropriate nutrition, way of life and more.

And more to the point, the majority of people are entirely uninformed of simply how unhealthy their existing regimen is for their brain. They have no idea that the things they're doing each and every single day are really harming their brains. And not just does this stop those individuals from executing efficiently every day; however, it might likewise cause a greater likelihood of Alzheimer's or dementia.

Simply imagine what you might achieve if rather than degrading and abusing your brain, you rather concentrated on nurturing it, training it and assisting it to grow. You may simply end up being limitless.

As discussed, many people have, at some time, demonstrated an interest in enhancing their physical strength and fitness. For this reason, many people have at least a basic idea of what physical fitness training involves and how to take care of their body's health.

However, seeing as brain health is a far less comprehended subject, this is a location that many individuals, in fact, do not have even standard understanding of!

This book then is going to act as a standard guide and intro to your brain, along with a sophisticated guide to how you can cultivate it and support it. We are going to cover all the things from the fundamentals of how the brain functions and great nutrition, all the way to far more advanced subjects like embodied cognition and smart drugs.

You are going to discover:

- How your brain functions

- The nature of intelligence

- How brain plasticity alters every little thing we once understood about the brain

- Why the appropriate nutrition is essential for optimal brain function

- The very best way of life practices for enhancing functionality and intelligence.

- How to boost concentration and focus

- How to train your body to train your mind

- How to utilize the best type of brain training to boost your cognition

- How nootropics work, who is taking them and whether you ought to participate

- Mental techniques such as CBT to assist your brain work for you

- The power of meditation

- How to enhance brain power by electrocuting it

- Main things you have to STOP doing to stay clear of harming your brain

- And A LOT MORE

By the end, you are going to have a far richer knowledge of your own brain and how to maximize it. Consequently, you can begin to enhance particular elements of your brain, in addition to its total function. This is going to have a substantial influence on basically every aspect of your life as you end up being more effective in social settings, less exhausted, more understanding towards others (and much better able to influence their thoughts and emotions), more in harmony with your own weaknesses and strengths and more.

When you find out how to update your own mental capacity, you can set off rapid improvements in every area of your life. Are you all set for that?

Chapter 1: How Your Brain Works

The brain is, without a doubt, the most effective computer on earth with billions upon billions of connections and near-limitless storage capability. There are still many things that we do not totally comprehend about our brains; however, we are beginning to comprehend increasingly more in time. And with each brand-new discovery comes brand-new methods to obtain more from our grey matter and update our effectiveness.

The bright side for you is that all this info is freely accessible now, and you do not need to go through years of complicated experiments and research study to uncover all the tricks. As a matter of fact, this chapter is going to act as a total guide to bring you up-to-speed on your brain.

However, a word of caution: this is intricate things. If you simply wish to get to the great things and begin finding out how to get more from your brain, then you can bypass this chapter. Nevertheless, I strongly advise that you do not, viewing as it is going to offer you a far greater understanding of what's really happening inside that skull of yours and consequently provide you more autonomy when it concerns finding brand-new methods to take advantage of your cranium's near-limitless capacity.

Nerve cells.

The initial thing to comprehend, then, is that your brain is comprised of billions of nerve cells. Nerve cells are 'brain cells,' and in a sense, they run much like any other cells within your body. They possess a cell membrane (the wall surrounding the cell); they have a soma (the body of the cell) loaded with cytoplasm, they have mitochondria to offer energy, and they have a nucleus, including your DNA.

However, brain cells likewise have a couple of 'additions.' Particularly, brain cells have dendrites and axons. The axons are the long 'tails' of your brain cells that extend from the back. The dendrites, on the other hand, are a lot like paths or tendrils that extend throughout the brain coming off of the soma. The task of the dendrites is to discover the axons of other cells, where they are able to then create a connection.

Nerve cells can be found in all sizes and shapes. While they are tiny, they are going to, in some cases, have connections extending all the way from one brain 'areas' to another to create connections. Brain cells do not really touch; however, they leave a little space referred to as the 'synaptic gap' and interaction then happens throughout that gap.

When a brain cell fires or illuminates, this is referred to as an 'action potential.' Throughout this point, a little electrical current leaps from the synaptic 'knob' over to one or a number of linking dendrites. This is the way signals navigate around the brain.

Each time a nerve cell fires such as this, it represents some type of subjective experience in the brain. For example, one location of the brain-- the occipital lobe-- offers vision. When nerve cells in this area fire, it triggers specs of light to resemble 'pixels' in the eyes of the audience. On the other hand, other nerve cells may make us remember a particular occasion, experience an odor, move a finger, or go to sleep.

Normally, nerve cells are organized into groups, which is what provides the brain unique 'areas' for a specific activity such as this. At any moment, you'll have a specific quantity of activity in various areas of the brain-- the whole brain is never ever illuminated concurrently. This is going to likely correspond with what you're thinking, seeing, and feeling at any time. And the connections indicate that seeing something is going to typically lead to you remembering another thing or deciding to do something.

Keep in mind that nerve cells just fire at one 'amount'. That is to state that there are no 'degrees' of firing-- a cell is either firing or it isn't. Nevertheless, it may need input from many various surrounding nerve cells prior to it ending up being excitable sufficiently to illuminate itself.

Hormones and Neurotransmitters

However, it is not simply a current that leaps across the synaptic gap throughout interaction in between cells. At the end of every axon at the synaptic knob are small 'sacks' referred to as 'neurovesicles.' These consist of neurotransmitters, that include the likes of serotonin, dopamine, and norepinephrine. Generally, a neurotransmitter is going to alter the excitability of your brain, the possibility of memories developing, your focus or your state of mind.

For instance, serotonin is the 'feel-good' neurotransmitter. This indicates that it is going to generally be launched when we see, consider or otherwise experience something that makes us pleased. It's likewise launched throughout a workout and when our body finds sugar!

On the other hand, dopamine is a neurotransmitter that gets launched when we believe something is vital. This then boosts focus, inspiration and the probability of a memory forming later.

Neurotransmitters, in this sense, inform us what we ought to be feeling about the experience of specific nerve cells firing. In many cases, a hormonal agent can imitate a neurotransmitter and vice versa. For example, testosterone has an impact on our brain cells, as does cortisol. Regularly, neurotransmitters just make a cell somewhat likely to fire an action potential, which leads to them being classified as either inhibitory or excitatory.

So as for neurotransmitters to have an impact on us, they have to communicate with 'receptors' situated on the dendrites of cells. To put it simply, a nerve cell may launch serotonin from its blisters when it fires; however, this is going to just have any influence on those linked nerve cells which contain serotonin receptors.

Neuroplasticity

In the past, researchers thought that the brain would be carved in stone after a specific age. To put it simply, it was believed that as soon as we matured, the brain would no longer keep on changing shape or grow, and all that is actually way off the mark. In truth, our brains keep on growing and altering practically constantly as we age, and this is how we are still able to develop brand-new memories and learn brand-new topics.

New brain cells can form in various areas of the brain, for example, by means of a procedure referred to as 'neurogenesis.' Simultaneously, brand-new connections can additionally be created and there is a basic rhyme to assist you in memorizing that: 'nerve cells that fire together, wire together.'

To put it simply, if you consistently hear a specific noise while experiencing a specific odor, you are going to ultimately get to the point where those 2 nerve cells form a connection. Gradually, that connection is going to end up being more powerful and more powerful through a procedure referred to as 'myelination.' Basically, the dendrites and axons associated with the connection end up being better insulated, which enhances the circuitry and renders it simpler for one nerve cell to induce the other to fire.

This is how we can wind up rote learning specific motions to the point where we no longer even have to consider them. One motion merely sets off the next motion immediately and nearly without our mindful input.

Comprehending brain plasticity-- likewise referred to as neuroplasticity-- is among the most crucial tricks to enhancing your brain function. This is the system through which all learning happens, and consequently, it could be used to learn a great deal of new skills and abilities!

Chapter 2: The Purpose of Our Brains

This standard guide has actually ideally provided you an excellent idea of how your brain functions on an everyday basis, and you're most likely currently seeing manners in which you can enhance its function: by boosting the amount of beneficial neurotransmitters, for instance, or by forming brand-new connections by consistently carrying out 2 actions together.

However, what can likewise assist, to a fantastic degree, is to comprehend what the brain was created for and thus why it is the way it is. And this all boils down to evolutionary psychology.

The most essential thing to comprehend about your brain is that it is created for survival. And how do you do that? By adjusting to your environment. Each and every single element of your brain function is connected to this standard concept, which implies that a great deal of the way your brain works could be anticipated in various scenarios.

At one point throughout the advancement of contemporary psychology, a field referred to as 'behaviorism' ruled. What this school of thought essentially said to us, was that every little thing could be rote learned and that our whole subjective experience of the world was based upon associations we created through our interplays with the world.

The most popular instance of this concept in action was the research study referred to as 'Pavlov's Dogs.' In this research study, Ivan Pavlov rang a bell every time he fed dogs. In time, he discovered that the dogs would establish a reaction to the noise of the bell-- they would start drooling even when there was no food present. This showed that they learned via association and that the repeating sufficed to create that association.

Behaviorism states that whatever we understand is found out in this way. As infants, we are mainly 'blank slates' (though not completely), and hence we find out how to connect with the world through association. For instance, we discover that by grabbing things, we are going to frequently be passed them. Therefore we establish an understanding of the reaching gesture. When we touch fire, it triggers a burning feeling, and the association that develops shows us not to touch flames once again. When we consume, it launches serotonin and we discover that we enjoy eating. We come to link the smell of cookies with granny's home, and we get to know the language by seeing how individuals respond to various words.

On a neural level, we now understand that this is all to do with neuroplasticity. And when something is really crucial (such as the fire), dopamine and other neurotransmitters are launched to make that memory develop even quicker.

Our environment is constantly altering, and hence this is the very best method for the brain to endure. By adjusting to various environments, our brains make sure that the habits we get are completely fit for the environment we remain in. Eventually, we find out how to stay clear of threats and gravitate toward food, shelter and sex.

Why is this so crucial to comprehend? Due to the fact that we're adjusting to any scenario we're placed in. That suggests that you're still adjusting today to operating in a workplace, being continuously stressed out and taking a look at your phone a lot. The connections you're not utilizing are atrophying, while lots of unhealthy habits keep on bolstering with time.

CBT and Embodied Cognition

However, while behaviorism did a great task of describing psychology for a long period of time, it was ultimately discovered to be excessively simplified and not able to describe the complete range of human experiences. For example, the majority of us would say that we can learn things by reading, for instance. How does this match the behaviorist system?

CBT (cognitive behavioral therapy) utilizes behaviorism as a beginning point, and after that, develops a cognitive component on top of that. This specifies that what we think likewise plays a crucial function—and that we can really produce brand-new associations by thinking. To put it simply, if you think of falling, then this can produce brand-new neural connections as if you were falling-- which consequently can cause the development of a phobia, or modifications in character.

Hold that idea in your head for a minute while we have a look at another idea: this one is referred to as 'embodied cognition.' Embodied cognition is a more current psychology theory that states all of our knowledge of the world around us originate from our bodies. This fits with the evolutionary description that our brains developed to assist us to endure in our environment based upon our interactions.

The question that was presumed to psychologists was this: when somebody says something to you, how do you comprehend that? You got to know English growing up, yes, however, what is it that enables you to comprehend English? Your brain does not innately comprehend English, so you need to be 'equating' that language into something such as a machine code so as to handle it. For some time, psychologists comprised the term 'mentalese' so as to describe this.

However, later on, a better theory was presented. Embodied cognition described that we comprehend language by connecting it back to our knowledge of the world around us. When you hear somebody saying to you a story about going through a chilly forest, you comprehend that by envisioning yourself going through a cold forest and this triggers all those appropriate neural connections to fire as you consider the ramifications of that, pertinent memories, and so on. And what's really taking place here is that the locations of your brain are firing as if that story was truly occurring to you. If you place somebody under an MRI scanner while you tell them about the time you swam, their brain regions are going to illuminate as if they were swimming.

And this is how just picturing something or imagining something can produce associations in your brain. In case you are high up and you keep picturing falling off that height, then your nerve cells are going to fire at the identical time as if you were falling off that height. This suffices to trigger those nerve cells to wire together and to develop a strong connection-- to the point where it's tough not to imagine falling off of that height. This triggers a flood of neurotransmitters associated with the experience of falling and you lose consciousness!

CBT is one thing you can utilize to develop more favorable connections and associations in your brain and we'll look more at how this functions eventually in the book.

Chapter 3: Brain Training

Comprehending all of this, it's simple to see how brain training can operate in theory-- by assisting you to produce more powerful connections throughout your brain and to produce brand-new connections totally-- thus learning brand-new abilities and enhancing those you have.

And this is what has actually brought about a great deal of brain training programs and websites that teach you to undertake things such as mathematics tests or memory challenges. The more you do this, the more you enhance those abilities and the much better your memory, attention or psychological arithmetic are going to end up being. So should you proceed and begin utilizing that sort of brain training? I say no.

While something such as Lumosity may be beneficial for challenging your recall or your spacial awareness, the truth is that they are far too particular to be all that beneficial in real life.

When you train yourself to end up being better at finding the variety of adorable penguins in a group, you end up being better at doing specifically that. You're reinforcing neural links around penguins. You're redoing that game repeatedly and ending up being better at that game-- however, this won't do much for your capability to consider responses in an interview. It's not transferrable to 'real-life' and because of that, it won't be very useful.

You understand what is an excellent way to train yourself to end up being better at interviews, though? Easy: subject yourself to more interviews! This is going to put you in the particular set of scenarios you need to have to boost that ability, and it is going to guarantee you're utilizing the right neural pathway. However, that's not to state that all brain training is a wild-goose chase ...

The Best Kind of Brain Training

The greatest kind of brain training there is, is merely to challenge yourself to carry out many various cognitive activities and to constantly expose yourself to unique challenges and scenarios.

Simply put, you have to regularly attempt brand-new things, regularly test yourself and push your brain to continue growing. The more you exercise your brain plasticity, the simpler it is going to be and the more dopamine, norepinephrine, brain-derived neurotrophic aspect, and so on, you are going to create.

It's just when you stop getting to know brand-new things and quit challenging yourself that your brain ends up being exceptionally un-plastic, and you start to lose skills.

Since brain plasticity can work both ways. A kind of 'pruning' does take place when you go for a long period of time without utilizing a particular neural path, which is why we are predisposed to forget things with time. What's more, is that the brain is going to ultimately stop creating neurotransmitters that improve neuroplasticity. Brain-derived neurotrophic factor (BDNF) and dopamine are connected to neurogenesis and myelination; however, if you never ever utilize them, they are going to happen less frequently. A healthy and delighted brain is a brain that you are utilizing in great deals of ways.

Consider what a fantastic learner you are as a child. Why is that? Partially, this is because of the reality that whatever around you is novel. The world is loaded with things you do not comprehend and the brain is flooded with neurochemicals so as to begin understanding all of it.

As you age, more connections are developed and you comprehend the world more. Nevertheless, you are going to still continue finding out great deals of brand-new things and experiencing great deals of brand-new things: as you head to college and school, as you move home, as you go through adolescence, when you discover how to drive, when you experiment with brand-new pastimes, and so on.

However, then you reach adulthood. You find a joyful relationship, you fall into a job you enjoy, and your life discovers a rhythm. You do that identical thing, every day for the following 40 years. And the older you get, the less brand-new experiences you expose yourself. You stick to the identical buddies, you stick at the identical pastimes ... and your brain stops developing.

And it's this that can ultimately result in danger as you end up being more likely to deal with age-related cognitive decrease or brain conditions like dementia or Alzheimer's. If absolutely nothing else, you end up being more absent-minded, more set in your ways and less capable to learn more. And this is one reason why fluid intelligence degrades as we grow older.

However, it does not need to be like that! Not if you comprehend how crucial it is to keep exposing yourself to brand-new things and to keep learning. Keep getting to know brand-new languages. Learn brand-new games. Link up with brand-new people. Experience brand-new locations.

Even simply remaining in a novel environment is going to trigger a flood of neurotransmitters connected with awareness and attention. Take various paths home from work! Opt for jogging and explore. And utilize your body-- learning with the body is actually what the brain is developed for, as we have actually seen, and therefore this is an exceptionally crucial method to keep challenging yourself and to keep learning.

Select activities that are going to teach your brain beneficial 'abilities' too. If you wish to get more from your brain, then why not get to know other languages to ensure that you have more methods to process information? Why not teach yourself to end up being better at mathematics?

Here's the paradox-- things such as this are going to really prove to be far more helpful in the real world than having a somewhat better memory anyhow!

Video Games Are Actually Good For You

What may shock you is simply how helpful video games can be in all this when it concerns enhancing your mental capacity. Once upon a time, we believed that video games were bad for kids-- that they would cook their brains and make them dangerous. The truth, nevertheless, could not be more different.

Video game have actually now been demonstrated in research studies to enhance choice making under pressure. Playing action shooters allows us to make better choices in less time than individuals who do not play video games. Simultaneously, they really enhance visual acuity-- they make us more effective at finding distinctions in color and at discovering things on the horizon (which naturally is an outcome of keeping an eye out for targets). Video games can even enhance your chances of 'lucid dreaming'-- a kind of dreaming where you understand you're sleeping and acquire the capability to control the contents of the dream and your movements!

However, that's not where the actual strength of video game lies. Rather, video games provide a really novel type of brain training due to the fact that each video game is various. Each video game utilizes various controls, which teaches us various motor abilities. And each video game presents us to brand-new 3D environments. In some cases, even physics is going to alter!

Each time you get a brand-new video game, you're pushed to learn the brand-new rules and controls. You need to begin discovering your way around a brand-new environment, and you need to alter how you think. This all takes plasticity as brand-new neural networks are created in your motor cortex, along with in your prefrontal cortex.

Each time you learn a brand-new video game, it resembles getting to know a brand-new skill. And you have the specific identical releases of dopamine when you get it right!

In fact, the fact is much more remarkable than that. Video games are addicting due to the release of dopamine. Why is dopamine launched when we play video games? Due to the fact that we're learning. The brain likes learning and if you can make that enjoyable, then all of a sudden, you'll begin progressing at anything!

Chapter 4: Should You Use Smart Drugs?

The last chapter has actually demonstrated to us that the very best method to enhance the brain actually, is simply to utilize the brain and to utilize it in great deals of novel situations and to practice things to improve at them. What a surprise! Reinforcing the brain needs practice and effort -- similar to reinforcing the body!

Absolutely nothing worth having comes easy, so they claim. However, this is going to appear like problem for a great deal of individuals (although I essentially just told you to play video game to get smarter). Sadly, a great deal of us do not wish to train our brains to get smarter-- we simply desire simple responses. This is the reason why 90% of individuals never ever wind up adhering to their training regimes! It's too tough-- they desire the body, self-confidence and strength; however, they do not wish to put in the work!

Usually, I would state 'too bad.' However, as it is, there might be a method to 'leap ahead' and get the outcomes you desire faster. And that is to utilize 'smart drugs.' Let's take a better look at this, how it functions, and whether it is for you.

What is a Nootropic?

A nootropic, likewise referred to as a 'smart drug,' is any kind of supplementation or medication that can make you objectively more intelligent in some capability. This may imply that you enhance your concentration, memory, your imagination, or something else. In either case, nootropics are to the brain what steroids and supplements are to the body.

However, are they safe? And do they work? That all depends upon what sort of nootropic you plan on utilizing! Today, reports inform us that approximately 90% of CEOs and executives throughout America are utilizing nootropics of numerous descriptions so as to get an edge on their competitors. These enable them to stay up later on, be more positive throughout presentations, and usually perform at their very best.

Among the most prominent types of nootropic to this end is modafinil. Modafinil is a nootropic that functions by increasing the quantity of a neurotransmitter referred to as 'orexin' in the brain. This neurotransmitter is at least partly responsible for controlling the brain's wake and sleep cycle, in addition to numerous other physical functions (such as hunger). Modafinil was initially developed as a method to deal with narcolepsy-- a condition that triggers individuals to go to sleep for no reason and without warning-- however it was discovered that it might likewise enhance numerous other functions such as attention, memory and reflexes. This is due to the fact that it can likewise increase dopamine, in addition to numerous other essential neurotransmitters. There are no recognized adverse effects, and the pill has a half-life of 10 hours. So theoretically, a CEO can pop one in the early morning and, after that, be more focused, alert, and less drowsy for an entire 10-hour day.

Another instance is Piracetam. Piracetam is a nootropic that boosts acetylcholine within the brain. Acetylcholine is a generic excitatory neurotransmitter within the brain, indicating it usually boosts the firing rates of nerve cells. This leads to the brain ending up being more alive, and subjectively, this may make you feel more alert, awake and more clearly familiar with your senses. Piracetam takes longer to work and needs to develop within your system in time-- however, a great deal of individuals discover the results really enjoyable with no noteworthy drawbacks.

On the other end of the spectrum, you have things such as 5-HTP. 5-HTP is 5 hydroxytryptophan, which is a precursor to tryptophan. Precursor implies 'building block'-- indicating that the brain utilizes these chemicals to create various other chemicals.

Serotonin is the feel-good neurotransmitter and is likewise rather repressive. All this implies that serotonin can assist in making you feel delighted and unwinded simultaneously and thus fight tension. Serotonin likewise converts into melatonin (the sleep neurotransmitter), which makes 5-HTP a beneficial sleep-aid when utilized prior to bed. A CEO may utilize something like 5-HTP to relax after a difficult day then, to carry out much better throughout a presentation by soothing nerves, or simply to sleep more deeply, resulting in a more efficient day the following day.

So should you utilize these sorts of nootropics? Naturally, this depends on you; however, as basic recommendations, the response would need to be no. There are no recognized negative effects for something such as Piracetam or modafinil; however, that is not to state that there are absolutely no problems. These compounds have actually not been evaluated for the long term, so nobody understands what would take place were you to utilize them over a ten years duration. Not just that, however, it's likewise a little worrying that we do not understand specifically how many of these nootropics function. 5-HTP we comprehend-- however; it's not known exactly how modafinil influence on orexin, just that it does. It's entirely unclear how modafinil attains its other benefits, on the other hand.

And while there are no 'main' negative effects, I can personally inform you that this isn't completely the case. It's well understood that modafinil is going to make you have to go to the toilet a great deal, while additionally reducing your hunger. This is obviously an outcome of it modifying the regulation of numerous physical rhythms. I additionally discovered that modafinil made me bite the interiors of my lips a lot, along with grinding my teeth-- most likely just an outcome of having great deal of stimulatory neurotransmitters playing around my brain.

Piracetam is going to offer you a headache unless you stack it with choline and many individuals discover that even then, they can wind up with both brain fog and headaches.

Some individuals have actually reported feeling long-term brain fog due to utilizing Piracetam.

Modafinil additionally makes me so concentrated that it isn't constantly a good idea. When I utilize it, I end up being 'glued' to whatever it is I'm doing. If that's work, terrific! I am going to then be entirely transfixed on work up until I wrap up. However, if I have a fast go on a video game prior to working, then there's a likelihood I'm not going to have the ability to stop. I'm going to finish that video game prior to getting any work done!

Similarly, crossing the street can end up being harmful as I discover myself so engaged in what I think that I can't appropriately take note of the street or to noises/movement in my environment.

I additionally discover it more difficult to be innovative, since a boost in norepinephrine and dopamine is really connected with a decline in creativity. We are at our most imaginative when we are unwinded since this enables our mind to 'roam.' The neuroscience behind this is that our brain is forming brand-new connections in between disparate nerve cells that would usually never ever be linked-- which is how innovation occurs. However, when you're extremely focussed, you end up being too focused on something and this hinders creativity.

The point of all this? The brain runs the way it does for a reason. Optimal brain function is not about having the ability to concentrate on something for a very long time. Optimal brain function has to do with having the ability to change from one brain state to another as required. You have to be extremely concentrated while you're working and after that, unwinded when you're not. You have to let your mind roam when you're attempting to come up with new ideas, and after that, concentrate when you're asked a hard question.

When you synthetically boost too much of a specific neurotransmitter, you make it extremely tough to do this, and you get 'caught' in one state. It feels optimal; however, as a matter of fact, it's simply a synthetic 'high.'

Another issue with these kinds of neurotransmitters is that they can, in fact, be addicting as a result of something referred to as 'tolerance and dependence.' What takes place here is that the brain adapts to that reduced or boosted neurochemical. For instance, if you have actually synthetically increased the quantity of dopamine in your brain on a routine incident, then your brain may react by eliminating dopamine receptors to make the brain less responsive to it. Additionally, it may decrease the quantity of dopamine you naturally generate.

In other words, you now require a larger dosage of the identical compound so as to get the identical sensation as in the past. And ultimately, your 'standard' can end up being so low that you feel bad up until you get it! While Piracetam and modafinil aren't formally expected to be addicting, 5-HTP, in fact, could be and is much better avoided because of this.

Neurotransmitters Do Not Exist in a Vacuum

As though all that wasn't sufficient reason, it's likewise crucial to acknowledge that neurotransmitters do not exist in a vacuum. That is to state that whenever you change a neurotransmitter, you are going to immediately have an influence on numerous others and have other impacts on the body. We have actually already seen, for example, that serotonin transforms into melatonin, and orexin impacts our bowel movements and appetite. Then there's the reality that serotonin links to hunger and that cortisol (likewise related to dopamine) impacts our testosterone levels.

There are certainly many neurotransmitters that we have yet to even find. And what this indicates is that when you take a nootropic that impacts one neurotransmitter, you're actually making all sorts of unknown modifications in your brain without actually understanding what the repercussions of that action may be. For this reason, it's extremely recommended to concentrate on other methods to get your psychological edge!

What About Caffeine?

However, there is a nootropic that the majority of us currently utilize regularly. That nootropic is obviously caffeine, which is the secret component in coffee and tea that makes us get up in the early morning and feel sharper. This is much like any other nootropic, the only distinction being that it has actually been around longer and is, for that reason, a bit more 'prevalent.'

So how does caffeine works? Essentially, caffeine has the ability to simulate a neurotransmitter in the brain, referred to as Adenosine. Adenosine is a by-product of the 'energy procedure' within the brain. When your mitochondria make use of glucose for energy, they carry this out by transforming it initially into ATP (adenosine triphosphate), and after that, splitting that ATP into parts ... consisting of adenosine!

Adenosine accumulates throughout the day, then as we utilize our brain cells for moving, thinking and powering our bodies. However, this compound is inhibitory and gradually makes us sleepier and exhausted. Ultimately, we end up being so slow that we're pushed to go to bed and a good night's sleep is then capable of clearing our brain of the unwanted adenosine.

What caffeine does is to obstruct the adenosine receptors. Since caffeine is a comparable shape to adenosine, it is able to plug the holes where adenosine is expected to go, which then stops adenosine from working its magic. This makes us feel more sharp and awake and triggers a surge in brain activity. This surge in brain activity then leads to a surge of other excitatory neurotransmitters being launched, which include norepinephrine, dopamine and more.

So is it safe to utilize? Is caffeine going to provide you a healthy kick? Yes and no. On the one hand, caffeine has really been demonstrated in research studies to decrease your odds of establishing Alzheimer's, and in that sense, it is neuroprotective. It does improve memory and wakefulness, and it's fairly really safe. Simultaneously though, caffeine is likewise basically 'stress in a cup.' It functions by increasing much of our stress hormones, and this can reduce imagination (as we have actually seen), while likewise triggering various other issues. More worryingly, caffeine is addicting owing to the systems we explained previously. If you end up being dependent on caffeine, you'll discover you can get raving headaches whenever you go for extended periods without it.

What's more, it has, in fact, been recommended that what much of us think of as 'early morning grogginess' is really simply a withdrawal sign from caffeine! Simply put, we get up and feel slow since we have actually gone for such a long time without caffeine!

It's actually up to you if you take it or not; however, this is an outstanding presentation of the dangers related to nootropics versus the advantages. My recommendation is to think about all these nootropics, such as laser tools. Keep away from them 90% of the time; however, when you definitely have to get a big quantity of work accomplished, think about utilizing one only for that day.

Chapter 5: Diet and Supplements

So, in general, the cons may simply exceed the pros when it concerns utilizing nootropic to reduce or boost amounts of particular neurotransmitters. However, that is not to state there's no chance you can efficiently boost your mental capacity with a little external support. The secret is just to change your focus to your long term brain health instead of attempting to get an instant increase to your intelligence.

And doing this is really easy with the eating plan. An eating plan is definitely important for brain health, and much of us do not recognize simply how vital it is in this regard. Let's have a look at simply a few of the nutrients and supplements that you can utilize to improve your mental capacity.

Amino Acids

Amino acids are the foundations of protein. When you consume any meat, your brain is going to break it down into the amino acids, and after that, recombine these to develop tissues around your body. These tissues include usage in the brain; therefore, taking in more amino acids could be utilized to really enhance the body's capability to grow and fix the brain!

However, this is not where the value of amino acids ends. Amino acids are additionally important for producing lots of neurotransmitters. For instance, l-tyrosine is utilized to develop dopamine, whereas tryptophan (gone over earlier) is utilized to produce serotonin. Others, such as l-theanine, can have direct impacts on the brain, and in this case, it's a rather soothing impact. L-carnitine, on the other hand, has an energy-boosting impact on the brain by boosting the efficiency of the mitochondria (more on this soon!).

As we have actually seen with 5-HTP, it is possible to take in much of these amino acids by themselves, so as to activate instant modifications in the levels of neurotransmitters. Nevertheless, this causes imbalances as we have actually found, and in spite of popular opinion, this is never ever a good thing.

So rather, the very best suggestion is to concentrate on attempting to get a healthy mix of as many amino acids as you can manage. By merely consuming a great deal of protein, or supplementing with amino acid items, it's possible to supply the brain with all the products it requires to develop all of the various neurotransmitters when it requires them. This then makes it greater at going into every frame of mind and guarantees that you can optimize your concentration, focus, relaxation and memory all simultaneously.

The very best method to easily get great deals of amino acids? To take in lots of eggs. Eggs are among the only 'complete proteins', meaning that they consist of all of the amino acids that the brain does not produce by itself. On top of this, they additionally include choline, which is the precursor to the excitatory neurotransmitter acetylcholine. They're a terrific source of healthy hydrogenated fat too, and viewing as the brain is primarily created from fat, this is additionally a really useful and crucial element.

Minerals and Vitamins

The identical goes for numerous minerals and vitamins. These, too, are utilized to produce a great deal of the neurotransmitters that are so extremely searched for by individuals attempting to improve their focus and productivity.

Vitamin B6 is particularly utilized to produce a big amount of neurotransmitters. Vitamin C, on the other hand, is crucial for boosting serotonin and enhancing the state of mind while likewise offering defense versus disease.

And there are lots of other functions for minerals and vitamins too. Vitamin B12 and iron both assist with blood circulation by creating more red blood cells. Vitamin D assists with the regulation of hormonal agents, specifically testosterone. Zinc plays an essential function in boosting neuroplasticity. Magnesium, on the other hand, assists in fighting anxiety and depression.

In other words, if you are not acquiring the micronutrients you require, then you are not providing your brain whatever it requires to work efficiently.

And this is why you have to stay clear of processed foods. Anything that is extremely synthetic such as a McDonald's hamburger or a bag of chips, is going to consist of calories to fill you up; however, it will not consist of the nutrients you require to operate. You'll survive; however, you'll feel worn out, slow and far less effective as a result.

Consume healthy salads, shakes and a great deal of veggies and fruit and you'll discover that you begin feeling sharp and healthier. The following best thing is a multivitamin, and if you get the right one of these, then it may do a whole lot to enhance the function of your brain in addition to your general wellness and health.

Vasodilators

If you're searching for an instant brain increase that you can obtain from foods and supplements, then search for vasodilators. A vasodilator is any compound that dilates the blood vessels (arteries and veins). These are going to permit more oxygen and blood to navigate the body, which consequently is going to lead to more arriving at your brain.

A specific favorite amongst nootropic-fans is vinpocetine due to the fact that this vasodilator concentrates on the brain particularly-- and the prefrontal cortex a lot more particularly. This suggests you're delivering more energy right to the part of the brain that you utilize for problem-solving and planning, and some individuals illustrate the sensation as a cold shower for your mind'.

Cognitive Metabolic Enhancers

This is an elegant phrase for anything that boosts your brain's energy levels, and typically, this suggests things that are going to boost the performance of your mitochondria. Mitochondria are the energy factories of your cells. They drift around within the cytoplasm, and they utilize ATP and glucose to power your physical functions-- consisting of brain function!

Various things can assist your mitochondria in carrying out much better and these consist of lutein, CoQ10, PQQ, l-carnitine and more. To put it simply, a mix of amino acids, minerals, vitamins and all types of lesser-known nutrients offered in supplement form.

Once again, the very best method is simply to consume a really well-balanced and healthy eating plan; however, you can likewise boost your energy levels even more by utilizing creatine. Creatine is a supplement that is extremely typically utilized by bodybuilders and athletes. Its primary function is to transform utilized ATP (ADP and adenosine) back into more useable ATP. To put it simply, it recycles adenosine, which thus supplies you with additional energy to utilize in your training.

The more recent surprise, though, is that this likewise boosts brain function by enhancing the energy effectiveness of brain cells. Essentially, it enables the brain to recycle its ATP too, which implies you get merely a moment or 2 of additional energy at optimum exertion. Research studies reveal that people who take creatine get a small increase to their IQ, so this is certainly a really reliable nootropic-- and one with absolutely no negative effects or dangers!

Creatine is created naturally in the liver and can likewise be acquired from your diet plan (sources like beef). Nevertheless, the very best method to see a substantial increase is to utilize it in supplement kind-- try to find creatine monohydrate.

Omega 3

Omega 3 fat is a fantastic anti-oxidant that is discovered in tuna and other oily fish, in addition to some nuts and different other sources. What makes omega 3 beneficial for the brain, however, is the reality that it can enhance 'cell membrane permeability.' Basically, this indicates that it makes the cell walls of the nerve cells simply a bit more permeable, thus permitting things to go through a bit more quickly. That consists of neurotransmitters, nutrients and more-- so it basically makes brain cells more receptive and thus offers you a small increase once more.

Anti-oxidants

Anti-oxidants are essential for caring for your brain's long-term health. These consist of omega 3, vitamin C, resveratrol and lots of other micronutrients.

Basically, anti-oxidants work by demolishing 'free radicals'-- compounds that harm cells when they enter contact with them and which can even result in cancer in case they make it through the nucleus and induce damage to the DNA!

Consuming anti-oxidants is, therefore, an extremely crucial technique for your total health and is going to likewise assist you in minimizing your possibility of disease by reinforcing your body immune system. Nevertheless, what we have an interest in today is how this can increase your mental capacity in the long run by safeguarding brain cells from damage and possibly decreasing your odds of establishing tumors later on in life.

Chapter 6: Other Options

However, what about plasticity? Can that be improved? We have actually currently seen a couple of approaches that can assist in enhancing plasticity. The initial one is to utilize your brain and to expose it routinely to novel stimuli. Similarly, we have actually seen that dopamine and magnesium benefit plasticity.

However, what about nootropics that impact this in a huge way? There are a number of choices out there as it occurs.

The initial nootropic that can increase plasticity is 'Lion's Mane.' This is a nootropic that acts straight on BDNF to boost the probability of brand-new connections being developed (and which boosts when we're presented with novel stimuli).

Lion's mane is really a mushroom and could be delighted in as a coffee. Once again, there's not a substantial quantity of details available concerning the underlying mechanisms or the long-lasting impacts; however, many individuals swear by this component as a method to get a psychological edge and some unequaled cognitive increases.

Another choice is to attempt CILTeP. This is a stack including a number of various natural nootropic compounds consisting of forskolin, l-carnitine, artichoke extract, and vitamin B6. The primary stars here are the artichoke extract and forskolin, which together boost 'cAMP' in the cells and consequently promote gene transcription. Suffice to state that it's expected to enhance long-term-potentiation (myelination), particularly, and some individuals discover it to be helpful without negative effects.

And after that, there's 'tDCS.' This means 'transcranial direct current stimulation' and essentially suggests that you are running a little current through your brain by means of conductive pads that are connected to your scalp.

The concept of tDCS is not to trigger your brain cells to fire, as there is inadequate electrical power being provided to the brain for that. Rather, it is just to potentiate them, to boost the quantity of BDNF, and to motivate plasticity. This has actually been shown to be helpful in many research studies, and there are once again no tested adverse effects. Pads are positioned in different ways around the head, which are called 'montages,' and these are developed to guarantee that particular brain locations get most of the current. This then alters the impact of the tDCS-- some montages make individuals more focused and alert while others can increase the state of mind or enhance sleep. What's especially intriguing is that the impacts appear to last about thirty minutes following usage.

Just as with more powerful nootropics, however, it is essential to exercise a little sound judgment here and to recognize that there's no such thing as a 'biological free lunch.' Apart from everything else, it's really difficult to know exactly the location of the brain that you're promoting simply by taking a look at an illustration of the scalp! And if you can boost learning in one location of the brain, you might, in theory, unintentionally trigger learning in other parts of the brain too that would be less beneficial. Proceed with care then!

However, with all that stated, this is absolutely a fascinating choice and particularly when you think about a) that there is a substantial quantity of proof recommending that this is a safe method to get a substantial brain increase and b) that there are numerous business items now offered that utilize this technology.

Chapter 7: Working With Your Brain

The appropriate nutrition can make a substantial distinction to your mental capacity then, and so can dabbling in nootropics and even tDCS provided that you're cautious with it.

Then there's the value of utilizing 'natural' brain training by stimulating yourself with great deal of brand-new challenges and experiences. However, in spite of all this, there is still one another approach that is even more reliable when it pertains to offering you an instant increase in your efficiency, cognitive function, and basically every element of your mental capacity. And that is to sleep more.

In case you are not obtaining a sufficient number of hours of sleep every night, then you are not executing at your finest, and it's that easy. This is due to the fact that you will still have an accumulation of adenosine in your brain, slowing you down, and since your brain really reinforces connections created throughout the day throughout the night. It's likewise while you sleep that you renew a number of your neurotransmitters, and in other words, this is a definitely important procedure for placing you back on top of your psychological game. Skip it, and you can anticipate feeling sluggish, absent-minded, slow and quite potentially even depressed.

Many people neglect this definitely vital aspect though and are going to continue to abuse their sleep-- attempting to work longer hours or get up previously. In the long run, this is going to harm your mental capacity and performance... so get to sleep.

Tips for Better Sleep

If you wish to enhance your sleep and therefore get up revitalized and much better able to concentrate on what you're doing, then follow these suggestions.

Take a Hot Bath

Having a hot bath right prior to bed is a wonderful method to prompt sleep. This is going to assist to unwind your muscles, and that makes it a lot simpler to sleep. In addition, however, it is going to likewise assist you to generate more sleep-related hormones and neurotransmitters and even to much better control your temperature level throughout the night, which likewise enhances your capability to be asleep.

Have a Bedtime

Another crucial idea is to head to bed at the identical time each night. Our bodies like routine since they are based mainly on rhythms. Our sleep rhythm is called the 'body clock' and is based not just on what time we wake up/go to bed; however, likewise on external signs like the weather and the sun.

If you go to sleep at the identical time each day, your body is going to begin to discover its natural rhythm to ensure that it's prepared to sleep when you are and not in the past.

Utilize a Daylight Lamp

You can likewise assist this procedure by providing yourself a 'daylight lamp.' This is a light that is developed to simulate natural sunshine by creating light with an extremely comparable wavelength. What's more, is that a daylight light could be set to begin slowly in the early morning to stimulate the ascending sun. Instead of being rudely 'shocked' awake, you'll rather be slowly poked by light.

Develop Your Environment

This is likewise why it's so essential to have thick drapes. If the light arrives in from outdoors, it can get to your brain through the thinner parts of your skull and set off the production of cortisol to wake you up. However, if you keep those drapes nontransparent, then you'll just have the light you set to inform your body when to get up.

Other crucial pointers are to have a peaceful area to sleep in and to make certain that your bed is as comfy as possible.

Cool off

Likewise, it is crucial to have a 'cool off' duration. This is an amount of time throughout which you're going to stay clear of anything that may stimulate you. That indicates you're staying clear of all types of tension; however, likewise, anything that simply wakes you up. So no video games, phones, or bright lights. The very best method to do this is to read something beneath dim light. Reading centers your internal monologue and thus stops your mind from roaming to difficult things. On the other hand, focusing on the text is going to make your eyes heavy, which likewise makes it simpler to drift off (and more difficult not to!).

Regimens and Rhythms for Your Brain

The reason this cool-down duration is so crucial is since it places you in an unwinded state prior to bed. This suggests that you'll have less excitatory neurotransmitters and more inhibitory neurotransmitters.

And this is a crucial idea to comprehend since, eventually, both your brain and your body are in one of two states: inhibited or excited. You are constantly either anabolic or catabolic.

Throughout the day, we change from being prepared for bed and drowsy and sharp and all set to go. When it gets dark, and we're tired by the end of the day, we have hints from the darkness, from the adenosine accumulation in our brain and even from supper (which triggers a production of sugar and melatonin/serotonin in the brain). Together, all this slows our breathing and heart rate, minimizes brain activity, and places us in a calm and creative mindset.

In the early morning, however, intense light triggers a surge of nitric oxide and cortisol in the brain, which 'boots us up.' Heading to work causes an increase of sound and colorful lights to discover their way into our brain and promote much more adrenaline/norepinephrine to wake us up even more. And it's by shifting in between these 2 states that the brain is usually able to constantly execute well.

The issue is that we're constantly sending out the incorrect signals or attempting to push ourselves to remain in one state too long. That's what takes place when we play loud computer game right prior to bed, or when we attempt and drive ourselves to work hard at 5 pm after we have actually just eaten.

A huge part of performing well is to comprehend the value of allowing our brain to go through its normal rhythms and attempting to collaborate with it to obtain the most from it.

And additionally, it is essential to attempt and stay clear of excess stress. Due to the fact that when you get too stressed out-- whether that is brought on by mental or physiological elements-- this, in fact, triggers us to end up being so concentrated that our prefrontal cortex completely closes down. This is a state referred to as 'temporal-hypofrontality.' While this could be a good idea often throughout sports, it's really the last thing you desire throughout a discussion or when you're attempting to be inventive!

CBT teaches us a great deal of methods we can utilize in order to conquer stress and put ourselves into the appropriate frame of mind for the task. These consist of visualizations strategies in addition to challenging ideas that may not be especially powerful. Meditation is additionally an exceptionally beneficial tool that you can utilize to attend to stress and place yourself in a much unwinded and calmer frame of mind when you have to.

Working Out

And lastly, it is definitely necessary that you work out a great deal if you wish to get the most out of your brain. Keep in mind; your brain is developed to assist you in adjusting and make it through in the environment by means of your physical interactions with it.

What's more, though, is that working out increases your memory according to research studies and promotes the production of many essential hormones and neurotransmitters. Even beyond this, working out is essential to enhance your blood circulation so that you may get more oxygen to your brain.

Conclusion of Brain Health 101

Congratulations on making it all the way here! We covered a great deal of complex subjects and actually did dive in deep when it comes to the processes of the brain and how to obtain the most from it. However, if you have actually made it to this point, then the excellent news is that you now have a far better understanding of how the brain functions than approximately 99% of the population.

And ideally, you can likewise now see the most effective methods to enhance your mental capacity through training, eating and through your way of life. Get a healthy eating plan, work out, expose yourself to new things, play computer games, get more sleep, and sometimes think about utilizing nootropics when you actually require a boost.

If you do all this and be aware of your rhythms and what's taking place inside your head at any time, then you are going to have the ability to take advantage of the type of mental capacity you never ever understood you had.

Natural Pain Management

Learn How to Achieve Pain Relief Naturally and Without Drugs so That You Can Live a Carefree Life Which We All Deserve

By Jim Russlan

Introduction to Natural Pain Management

Pain is an unavoidable truth that a large number of individuals everywhere throughout the world live with each day of their lives. For some, who are in chronic pain, this is something they need to live with each waking second, which is probably going to make life entirely insufferable.

The truth of the matter is that we all, are either acquainted with pain or will have moments of pain sooner or later. Does this accordingly imply that we need to embrace pain as an unavoidable truth?

The uncomfortable response to the question is most likely yes, except if you live in a cotton-fleece lined casing for each moment of existence, it is practically unimaginable to stay away from the sort of mishaps that unavoidably cause pain and distress. Nonetheless, in a circumstance like this, the pain is typically brief and regardless of how intense it may be at the time, it passes decently fast.

In the event that you trap your finger in the entryway or smack yourself on the back of the hand with a hammer, indeed, it hurts like heck and the pain will be painfully exceptional, of that there is no question.

In the event that you tumble off your bicycle and split your knee, it hurts and getting an unexpected kick or smack as you are participating in sports does not hurt any less just because of the fact that your buddy didn't intend to inflict the pain.

By definition, intense pain of this sort typically passes and while catching your finger in the entryway or tumbling off your bicycle can leave a mark that hurts for a couple of days, it is, in any case, still a moderately brief painful circumstance that you are in. However, these are additional times when relief from pain is something that you will most likely look for, due to the fact that the essential truth is that humankind, by and large, isn't truly adept at managing pain without some sort of outside assistance.

If you have a knee or finger that hurts for a few days, envision how much more insufferable it would be needing to live with constant pain, the chronic pain that bothers you during every single moment of your life. In the event that you are one of the lucky ones who was never unlucky enough to endure chronic pain, it is likely difficult to envision a circumstance where the pain is consistent in your life, yet there are many individuals for whom this is their regular reality.

Obviously, through the span of the previous century since Felix Hoffman figured out how to create a stable variant of acetylsalicylic acid, otherwise called aspirin, man has created numerous painkillers that are utilized by millions everywhere throughout the world every single day.

A large number of these medications are truly viable as painkillers; however this does not change the fact that, similarly as with all chemical-based pharmaceuticals, there are potential symptoms linked to a significant number of these medications.

There are individuals who can't ingest these medications as well, individuals who are either allergic to them or are taking different prescriptions which disallow them from taking specific sorts of painkillers.

For instance, for a great many individuals everywhere throughout the world who ingest anticoagulant tablets like heparin or warfarin sodium daily, aspirin is a distinct impossibility as it also can be a blood thinner.

Along these lines, while not dismissing the viability of using painkilling drugs, there is a shocking number of individuals who can't utilize chemical-based painkillers. Also, there are a large number of individuals who would prefer not to utilize chemical-based analgesics (painkillers) since they comprehend that therapeutic science isn't flawless and that while most of the symptoms of most ordinarily utilized painkillers are well-known, there likely could be side effects that have not yet been found.

There are consequently many individuals who are searching for natural methods for managing their pain. This guide is going to give you a wide range of pain management options that are natural so that on the off chance that you pursue the natural course to dispose of your pain, you know about the choices and the potential drawbacks of various different methods for dealing with pain.

Chapter 1: Explaining Pain

The word pain can be utilized from numerous points of view, so it is presumably worth explaining what precisely we mean by the word pain with regards to this book.

All through this guide, I am talking about physical torment pain, unlike the sort of general life-enveloping enduring pain that can make each day into a drudgery. The sort of pain we are discussing here does not, for instance, incorporate the sort of suffering that you may endure on the off chance that you have no cash or are without a roof over your head, emotional pain expedited by family deprivation, etc.

As we have all felt physical pain now and again, we as a whole comprehend what it is, nevertheless finding a precise definition is, in reality, far harder than it may from the outset seem like it ought to be.

For instance, while the International Association for the Study of Pain characterizes it as 'an unpleasant emotional and sensory experience associated with actual or potential described damage', it is necessary to comprehend that pain is mostly subjective.

What one individual would consider a horrifying agony could be just a minor aggravation to another person, and individuals who experience the ill effects of chronic pain each day forget about it somewhat despite the fact that the pain does not leave.

Hence, it is now and again proposed that the definition given by a prominent pain management specialist Margo McCaffrey in 1968 may be seen as increasingly precise. She said that 'pain is whatever the experiencing person says it is, existing whenever he says it does.'

What is absolutely unquestionable is the truth that practically 50% of visits to specialists and medicinal professionals in the USA consistently are because of a pain issue that the patient needs handling. At the point when this occurs, your doctor is going to do the following.

Right off the bat, they are going to attempt to describe the pain itself utilizing different various criteria or portrayals, for example, magnitude, kind of pain(dull, throbbing, etc.), the cause behind the pain and its location.

In the wake of posing these questions, if there is no unmistakable cause behind the pain, they will analyze you to discover why you are enduring what you are as there is obviously some fundamental explanation behind your pain of which you are not completely mindful.

As a rule, the pain is going to leave with basic medications like rest, and obviously, pain-relieving prescriptions. In any case, we have just observed that numerous individuals endure ceaseless chronic pain, a torment that turns into another medical issue in itself and does not leave voluntarily or because of medicines.

Pain is a basic piece of the body's survival mechanism, a characteristic reflex response instructing you to back off from something that can possibly harm you. Moreover, it additionally helps you to modify your actions with the goal that whatever it was that caused you pain is not done again, accordingly securing you against further physical mischief or harm.

Pain is a very acute sensation – once in a while we are excessively aware of it, and it can strike whenever, anyplace, either because of a horrendous accident or on account of the abrupt or progressive beginning of an unanticipated medical issue.

Chapter 2: How It All Starts

it is, by and large, accepted that when we are born, each individual has a working natural pain control system.

Besides, it is set that in our prehistoric days, these pain management procedures or chemicals (hormones, catalysts and other regular chemicals in the body) would be activated nearly from birth on the grounds that the need to guard against pain and danger was much more prominent back then.

All things considered, and, after it's all said and done, millions of years ago, our forerunners felt pain, yet they didn't have medicine that they could take to dispose of it when the pain struck. While some recommend that natural solutions for help with pain and discomfort date from these days, it is still true that individuals in those days had far fewer options for successful relief from pain accessible, thus the conviction that natural pain management instruments were undeniably more pervasive.

This is essential to comprehend on the grounds that later research has added to this by showing that these regular components have not vanished completely.

In any case, the world that an infant lands in is these days an altogether different world to that of our cave-dweller ancestors back in the day. Consequently, there is some proof that modern life just falls shorttt to 'switch on' these regular pain control procedures.

This was featured in an examination at the University of Maryland in Baltimore, that demonstrated that suckling and sugar initiate these characteristic pain management procedures in youthful infants. Besides, they additionally concluded that these control procedures appear to have something to do with the spinal segment, in spite of the fact that the examination was not performed on people. The definite correlation of this to people has still to be determined with any level of conviction.

In any case, the examination proposed that a couple of minutes of suckling and sugar water administration to infants could essentially diminish the degree of pain felts a couple of moments after the fact.

This is a significant bit of knowledge for any parent who is expecting as it proposes that from the day that child is conceived, it is conceivable to develop their natural protection from pain reasonably rapidly and effectively.

While there plainly should be more examination on this, it is unquestionably something to be aware of on the off chance that you are a parent or you see yourself as becoming one soon.

Chapter 3: Analgesic Options

Over the counter painkillers

Ibuprofen is currently one of the most generally utilized pain-relieving analgesics and as you can purchase this medicine in practically any store, it is a drug that a huge number of individuals everywhere throughout the world use when they are dealing with minor pain, for example, a headache or some other comparable condition.

Actually, aspirin is a non-steroidal anti-inflammatory drug and was the main medication of its sort to be found and isolated. For most of the individuals, this medicine is a moderately safe option to take, despite the fact that as recently recommended, it is a medication which should be kept away from individuals who are as of now taking different prescriptions with which it shouldn't mix.

What's more, it is assessed that around 1% of individuals experience the ill effects of an aspirin hypersensitivity, which is most ordinarily observed on the skin as hives, swellings and rashes. An aspirin hypersensitivity can expedite asthma episodes in individuals who are prone to asthma, with an expected 10% of asthma sufferers prone to endure this type of unfavorably susceptible response to aspirin. This can stretch to forming into anaphylaxis in the worst-case scenario.

Aspirin can likewise cause upset stomachs and loose bowels, just as hemorrhage and bruises because of its anticoagulant properties.

In an exceptionally modest number of cases, aspirin can prompt Reye's Syndrome, which is a conceivably deadly condition portrayed by damage to numerous inside organs, particularly the brain and liver. Given the magnitude of this specific condition, early detection of Reye's Syndrome is significant since it could result in brain damage or death.

Reye's disorder goes through five unmistakable stages, with the first being described by overwhelming vomiting that isn't turned around by eating, general lack of energy, bad dreams, and all-round disarray. In the event that any individual who is taking aspirin shows any of these side effects, it is totally vital to get them to a specialist or a clinic as fast as could be expected under the circumstances.

Paracetamol is another broadly utilized and by and large accessible pain-relieving analgesic which is also powerful for decreasing fever too. Therefore, it is generally utilized as a treatment for migraines, fever, and all manner of pains and aches.

Paracetamol is, in fact, known as an aniline analgesic and is still generally utilized for the treatment of pain since all other comparative analgesics were pulled back as it is accepted that they contribute to cancer development (which up until this point, paracetamol does not). Nonetheless, the way that it is produced using coal tar may give you some reason to scrutinize this, as carbon is frequently accepted to have cancer-causing characteristics too.

In ordinary dosages, one of the benefits of paracetamol is that it doesn't disturb the stomach lining or influence blood coagulation.

In any case, higher than prescribed utilization has been believed to have a potential association with gastrointestinal bleeding and high measurements have the ability to cause liver harm, which can be deadly in the most extreme cases. Without a doubt, paracetamol poisoning is the main source of intense liver shutdown in most Western nations and it is the manner in which the vast majority of people end it all in these nations.

Moreover, a big study led in 30 nations and including more than 200,000 youngsters in 2008 and published in the main medicinal publication 'The Lancet' found that the utilization of paracetamol in the initial year of life made kids unquestionably bound to create asthmatic symptoms at around age six or seven. What's more, kids who took paracetamol during the initial year of life, and furthermore youngsters who took the medication at ages 6-7 exhibited a far higher probability of developing skin inflammation and rhinoconjunctivitis later as well.

Ibuprofen (Nuprin, Advil and so on) and Naproxen (Aleve) are both NSAID resembling aspirin. They subsequently share a whole lot of the potential symptoms that have just been featured as being endemic to aspirin. For example, aspirin hypersensitivity, agitated stomach and a greater danger of asthma episodes can be similarly credited to both of these prescriptions as they can to aspirin.

Aspirin conveys extra dangers as it is accepted to boost the danger of myocardial infarction (heart attack) whenever taken in high doses and you can likewise cause or compound IBS, Crohn's disease and ulcerative colitis because of its capacity of beginning the process of gastrointestinal bleeding.

With Naproxen, the most generally revealed reactions are diarrhea or constipation, sluggishness, irritated stomach, stuffy nose, and acid reflux.

In any case, while the NSAID's are probably going to have a slight boost in probability for strokes and heart attacks, the hazard related to Naproxen could be even more alarming. In fact, the National Institute of Health ended a trial into the impacts of Naproxen as a medication for diminishing the seriousness of Alzheimer's as a result of the assumption that the medication essentially boosted the possibility of stroke or a heart attack.

Since that time, further investigation proposes that at ordinary measurements, the expanded danger of enduring stroke or a heart attack is genuinely low in spite of the fact that, as you will find in the following segment, this is unquestionably not valid for all NSAID's.

Prescription Drugs

As a general perception, the majority of the pharmaceutical painkillers that are recommended by specialists can be categorized nto one of two classifications.

The primary category is comprised of more potent non-anti-inflammatory drugs than those that are accessible over the counter, for example, ibuprofen and aspirin.

The second category is comprised of medications that your doc may give to manage your pain are the opiate or synthetic opiate-based drugs. How about we begin with a handful of the more typical NSAID's that your primary care physician may endorse.

Celecoxib (Celebrex), Tramadol (Ultram), Diclofenac (Naklofen, Volteran, Arbitren, and so on) and are largely NSAID's that carry with them the typical array of symptoms of consuming medications of this nature, for example, an expanded danger of bleeding on the inside and on the outside, bruises, upset stomachs, diarrhea and constipation and so on.

In any case, not at all like Naproxen with which it currently seems that the possibility of the expanded danger of enduring a heart attack or stroke at ordinary dose is little, the hazard is fundamentally higher with both Diclofenac and Celecoxib. Moreover, the risk is, by all accounts, expanded independently of the dose in spite of the fact that, obviously, the risk will increase as your dose is expanded.

Research shows that the expanded heart attack and the stroke risk factor is 1.62 contrasted with non-users. This shows an expanded risk that numerous chronic pain sufferers will endure as an end-result of the more prominent pain management of these medications in contrast with less potent medications, for example, aspirin. Basically, it appears that many pain sufferers know the expanded dangers and are eager to live with them to dispose of their pain.

Also, the danger of enduring kidney or liver harm seems, by all accounts, to be expanded with each of the three medications incorporated into this category and should such harm happen, it seems that, as a rule, it is probably going to be irreversible.

Vicodin, Demerol and Lorcet are all options that depend on synthetic or natural opiate-based drugs that are utilized to treat different distinctive ailments and pains brought about by these conditions.

Demerol is a medication that contains pethidine, which for most of the twentieth century was the most generally supported opiate-based medication, with 63% of specialists recommending it for intense pain and 22% endorsing it for chronic pain in 1983. The fame of the medication originated from the notion that it should be safer while additionally being more potent than morphine-based medications, which were the main option accessible at the time.

Since that time, be that as it may, this has been demonstrated to be false. Without a doubt, due to the brief length of its effectiveness and low potency, it is questionable whether Demerol was ever successful by any stretch of the imagination.

Then again, it conveys an unquestionably higher risk of causing neuropathological issues, for example, wooziness and seizures, as opposed to numerous other contending drugs. Consequently, it is not endorsed all that often these days. Truth be told, a few nations, have either put extreme limitations on the utilization of Demerol or restricted it through and through.

The symptoms of Vicodin are luckily not as serious as those of Demerol, with the most widely recognized being nausea, upset stomach, discombobulation or dizziness. In uncommon cases, Vicodin can cause hypersensitive responses, jaundice, unconsciousness, bruises, bleeding, clogging and changing sex drive; however, these are the special cases, as opposed to being the norm.

One Vicodin issue that is noteworthy is the fact that it is a medication to which it is quite easy to develop tolerance to. Thusly, numerous individuals are enticed to take bigger portions of Vicodin with an end goal to battle the impacts of expanding familiarity with the medication, which will normally diminish its adequacy.

While expanding the dose along these lines will battle the pain all the more rapidly and all the more viably, all sedative based medications are addictive and clearly, the greater amount of them you take, the more rapidly, all things considered, you become dependent. Vicodin can be profoundly addictive because of the hydrocodone yet while expanding the rate at which you take the medication to mitigate your pain is going to work, the harming impacts in both medicinal and social terms could be incredibly unsafe.

Getting to be dependent on Vicodin is a classic instance of being dependent on professionally prescribed medications and despite the fact that this is an endorsed medication, this does not reduce its consequences. For instance, reports of noteworthy legal and social issues for Vicodin addiction sufferers are regular as they visit a great many specialists after specialist to attempt to get a remedy to nourish their increasing appetite.

The 'potential antagonistic symptoms' of Vicodin in this way go way past the transient physical or medicinal reactions featured before. They incorporate numerous undeniably harmful symptoms which can and will unfavorably influence your quality of life on the off chance that you become dependent on this specific medication.

Keep in mind, all opiate-based medications are normally addictive so you should consistently apply a lot of alertness to any medication of this sort. As proposed, the compound in Vicodin that makes it so addictive is hydrocodone, Lorcet is among the brand names that are linked to this very drug.

That is why this medicine, in particular, is so addictive. Those who are addicted suffer from a lot of liver problems. Overdosing on Lorcet or any similar medicine based on hydrocodone can cause respiratory depression, heart issue, seizures, jaundice, amnesia, blackouts and ultimately death.

A lot of opiate-based drugs incorporate acetaminophen, which means that even a slight overdose can cause jaundice or any kind of serious liver damage which can't be reversed.

To sum it all up...

Potential side-effects are present in all pharmaceutical analgesics and these side-effects range from mild such as diarrhea or upset stomachs all up to serious problems which can't be reversed such as the failure of heart or liver, and even death.

Keep in mind that the worst-case scenario won't be the reality for most people who take chemical-based pharmaceutical analgesics. Still, it is undeniable that if one person out of hundred goes through an allergic reaction because of the aspirin or if someone finds out that their asthma was made worse because of the drug, the chances of enduring the mentioned side-effects go way up.

Taking everything into consideration, there are a lot of reasons to steer clear of these drugs and that brings us to the consideration of the available alternatives. Luckily for all of us, alternative options are abundant and anyone who is looking for natural pain management options will find something for them. That is what the remainder of this book is all about.

Chapter 4: What Kind of Pain Are You Dealing With?

Before your doctor prescribes any kind of pharmaceutical analgesic, it is very important to consider what kind of pain you are suffering from. First, they will try to determine whether you are dealing with something acute or chronic and whether there is some kind of circumstance or condition which is behind the pain before any kind of decision about the medicine is made.

If you are buying over-the-counter painkillers, the situation isn't all that much different since even though fever and pain from a headache can be dealt with effectively by taking Tylenol or paracetamol, using aspirin would prove a lot less effective for handling the fever issue.

Comparative considerations apply when you are seeking natural pain management options in light of the fact that some options are going work better in some painful circumstances than they would in others. Besides, in the event that you have a particular ailment or circumstance that is causing pain, some natural pain management options are probably going to be more suitable than others.

For instance, the painkilling approach that you utilize to dispose of spinal pain or a headache is probably going to be fundamentally different to the methodology that you embrace on the off chance that you are attempting to battle the pain brought about by cancerous growth or it's treatment or the pain related with labor and pregnancy.

Consequently, a significant number of the options that will be disclosed are probably going to be more compelling in specific conditions or circumstances than in others. You have to realize what sort of pain it is that you have to deal with before settling on the ideal method for utilizing natural pain management options and strategies to limit the side-effects of your issues.

Chapter 5: Pain Relief Through Massage

There are more than 80 distinct styles of massage and body treatment, a significant number of which have been created by individual experts who have taken the first massage idea and created it because of their practical encounters.

Moreover, there are many related practices like shiatsu and reflexology , which are extensively related yet not so much synonymous with the massage that a few people now and then mistake for massage.

The fundamental idea of massage as a technique for relieving pain is that rubbing various spots of your body confounds or 'diverts' capacity to notice the pain due to what is known as the 'gate control theory'.

This hypothesis depends on the idea that pain driving impulses travel from different spots of your body through the central sensory system and your spinal column to the brain. It is just when these pain signs land in your mind that you register pain despite the fact that obviously, it involves an extremely modest number of nanoseconds between the signals occurring at some spot on your body and your cerebrum feeling pain.

The 'gate control theory' clarification of why massage functions as help with pain management methods is based upon the idea that your body just can send a limited number of stimuli to your mind at any one time, and if the certain stimuli don't arrive at your cerebrum, they won't be processed. Therefore, when you are getting a kick out of an enjoyable massage, the stroking sends other progressively pleasurable stimuli to your mind, accordingly 'populating' the nerves that convey these signals with a positive message ruling out the negative, painful message.

There is additionally some proof that pleasurable massage brings about the arrival of endorphins, which are chemicals created by the pituitary gland, the constructive outcomes of which are similar to impacts of opiate medications. In any case, as endorphins are totally normal and their generation is carefully constrained by your body, there is no potential mischief engaged with encountering the bliss or elation that is frequently known as an 'endorphin rush.'

Moreover, endorphins additionally counteract nerve cells from discharging more pain signals, which is, for instance, one reason why top sports players can regularly keep on contending even when they are injured, in light of the fact that extraordinary movement combined with excitement prompts the 'rush' that blocks the pain.

Coming up next are the types of massage that are usually connected with providing relief from discomfort.

Swedish Massage

Swedish massage is a style that was first created in Scandinavia about 200 years ago by Pehr Henrik Ling who learned a considerable lot of the essentials that he would later form into Swedish massage from a Chinese individual named Ming with whom he sailed for a long time.

After he came back to Copenhagen, he built up these ideas still further into something like what we perceive as Swedish massage, which was first brought to the USA during the 1850s.

From only a little bunch of Swedish massage centers in Washington and Boston, they would now be able to be found in pretty much every town and city all through the USA (and all through most other western nations also). Henceforth, Swedish massage is the most favored type of massage in the USA and if utilizing this sort of massage to bring help with discomfort seems like something which may work for you, it ought to be moderately simple to locate a neighborhood professional.

The fundamental idea of Swedish massage is that it centers around long, skimming strokes of the masseuse hands over your skin, with some 'kneading' (precisely the same activity as though you were making bread) applied to the use of friction strategies to the most problematic muscle areas.

Most generally, most of the strokes go towards the heart, following the bloodstream on the grounds that there is an emphasis on rejuvenating blood flow through the delicate tissues. This type of massage can be performed in a generally fiery and not all that delicate way or it can be extremely delicate and soft, contingent on conditions and necessities.

Swedish massage is generally used to provoke a wide scope of good things:

• It helps with muscle relaxation. Therefore, if there is a muscle pain because of tension, stress or muscle damage, muscles can be loosened up by the massage, which can reduce the swelling and pain.

• It can decrease the pain from other substantial harm, for example, breaks, sprains, sciatica, hardened joints and strains. This applies similarly to individuals who have endured injuries and to the individuals who are getting older and feeling the effects of that!

• There are substances in the body that normally hinder the recuperating from muscle sprains, strains and damage. Since Swedish massage is successful for expelling lactic and uric acid (and other waste) from your muscles, it accelerates the recuperation procedure, implying that any pain you are enduring will vanish all the more rapidly.

• As Swedish massage can be utilized to stretch muscles, ligaments and tendons, it forestalls the sort of damage that may cause pain sometime in the future. As a result, Swedish back rub isn't just corrective, but preventive as well.

• When all is said and done, Swedish massage aids blood flow, loosens up the nerves and invigorates the nervous system. It likewise diminishes pressure and strain which can be a reason for physical pain as rigid and tense muscles are undeniably bound to endure pain or damage instead of the muscles that are adaptable and loose.

Basically, 95% of individuals who experience Swedish massage leave their session feeling especially better in a wide range of ways, both mentally and physically.

The advantages of Swedish massage for any individual who is enduring any of the specific sorts of pain featured previously are evident. On the off chance that you are enduring muscle, joint or sprain pains, attempting Swedish massage before turning to pain-relieving analgesic makes all the sense in the world.

So, to locate a neighborhood Swedish massage parlor, the best tool to utilize is Google maps to discover what you're searching for. You will likely get a lot of results by typing in Swedish massage along with the name of your town in the search bar. Still, there is no doubt that you would find a lot of good results even if you were to search for something less specific such as massage even though the results would be a lot less precisely targeted.

Deep Tissue Massage

As the name would presumably imply, the idea of deep tissue massage is to work the muscles more thoroughly than what is expected in the case of Swedish massage, with a definitive target being the release of deep muscle strain to lessen potential muscle stress and pain.

Utilizing this specific type of massage, the masseuse is going to typically utilize direct pressure or friction aligned with moderate strokes as a method for 'burrowing' further into the muscle filaments and tissues to mitigate the deepest tension. This isn't to propose that deep tissue massage has to hurt, yet it is definitely more observable than Swedish massage, as far as the beneficial effects are concerned.

With this specific system, the movements are most regularly done over the muscle filaments in a 'cross-grain' pattern and administered with the fingers, thumbs or maybe in some cases, even elbows. Along these lines, the impacts are probably going to be most valuable to the individuals who have deep muscle pressures, strains and tensions that are the reason behind their pain or uneasiness. Thusly, if Swedish massage does not give you the help with discomfort that you were hoping for, it may be a good idea for you to consider going one step further with deep tissue massage.

Thai Massage

It was initially accepted that the beginning of
Thai massage was in India where it was
intensely affected by Ayurvedic ideas and
reasoning before moving to Thailand around
2500 years prior.

The first massage techniques that originated
from India have been progressively affected by
customary Chinese drugs which means that what
we presently perceive as Thai massage can be
described as a physical indication of a blend of
the two extraordinary medicinal conventions of
the East.

With the first predecessors of Thai massage
originating from India, you probably will not
find it surprising that this specific type of
massage is regularly called Thai Yoga Massage,
as certain individuals depict it as a yoga session
without doing the activity of yoga yourself.

It is a type of massage that is extensively more empowering and demanding than Swedish massage for instance, which obviously implies that on the off chance that you endure genuine physical issues of any kind, you ought to counsel with your primary care physician before thinking about giving Thai massage a shot.

The back rub itself is generally performed while the 'guest' is on the floor and includes the masseuse utilizing their hands, legs, feet and knees to perform the massage. In a comparable (however unique way) to deep tissue massage, Thai massage gets down to even deeper degrees of your joints and muscles, giving relief that you simply won't get from Swedish massage.

Individuals who have experienced Thai massage will disclose to you that it is both inconceivably unwinding and empowering at the very same time, and that muscle pains and aches and discomfort are going to leave after the underlying 'buzz' has died down.

On the off chance that you have muscle pains and you aren't happy with the results of Swedish massage, this is another option to think about.

Chapter 6: Acupuncture

Acupuncture is an old Chinese practice that had been performed for many years, one that has been demonstrated on numerous events to be amazingly viable for advancing general wellbeing and for diminishing various sorts of pains.

The primary thing to comprehend about acupuncture is that it embraces an all-encompassing perspective on any mental or medical issues that you may endure, including physical pain.

Fundamentally, while a Western specialist will treat the manifestations of the pain by recommending a medication that deals with just the zone where the pain is felt, an acupuncturist holds the view that the 'something' that has caused your pain isn't really situated in that specific part of the body. Subsequently, they are going to attempt to discover the underlying driver of that pain in whichever place that might be situated in your body before managing it.

Acupuncture depends on the idea that each person contains an 'essential vitality' stream that courses around their body and that pains, ailments or afflictions are signs that this crucial vitality stream has been disturbed somehow. Vitality streams along meridians or 'channels' that are perceived by acupuncture to associate certain clearly detached pieces of the body to each other.

Hence, when an issue that can be seen as a disturbance in the crucial vitality stream shows up, it makes sense that the acupuncturist is going to address that issue by endeavoring to open up the proper vitality meridian with the goal that the stream can be reanimated and the issue resolved.

There are locations along every one of these meridians or channels that are perceived by Chinese acupuncturists as being 'acupoints', the spots where intrusions most normally happen. Henceforth you have the procedure where the conventional acupuncturist are going to insert extremely fine, long needles through the skin to invigorate these 'acupoints' to free up the stuck vitality stream.

These days, numerous conventional acupuncturist still proceed with the act of utilizing needles yet there are numerous elective types of acupuncture, for example, utilizing little, focused electrical charges on the equivalent 'acupoints' as a method for reanimating the vitality stream. Different experts have been known to utilize magnets while there is continuous development and study of utilizing lasers for similar purposes.

One of the issues with acupuncture is that while it has been utilized for more than 2000 years as a treatment for pain and sickness, it is still not completely comprehended why acupuncture functions just as it does. Albeit even medicinal specialists acknowledge that needle therapy can be an all-around profoundly successful treatment for managing pain, we despite everything, don't generally comprehend why it is so.

There are numerous hypotheses advanced concerning why acupuncture can be such a viable treatment for pain in obviously detached regions of the body. One of these speculations proposes that acupuncture points invigorate the central sensory system, which at that point discharges hormones and chemicals into the muscles and spinal column.

It is additionally suggested that these hormones and chemicals adjust the experience or view of pain while likewise animating the body's capacity to recuperate itself significantly more rapidly than what would be the case without acupuncture. Consequently, the relief from discomfort is increasingly prompt and as the fundamental condition is managed all the more rapidly, the agony subsides unquestionably more quickly as well.

Another hypothesis propounded by Western researchers is that there is some proof that acupuncture points serve as bodies electromagnetic 'intersections.' Subsequently, by reinvigorating the intersections, it opens up the progression of electromagnetic charges all through the body, which thus seems to animate the progression of normal painkilling chemicals, for example, endorphins.

Different examinations have demonstrated that acupuncture seems to adjust the chemistry of the brain by inciting the creation of neuro-hormones and neurotransmitterrrs. Furthermore, in light of the fact that it seems as though acupuncture reanimates inconspicuous changes in your central nervous system's capacity to manage pain, there seems to be some proof for why acupuncture is by all accounts such a successful treatment for pain.

One of the wonders of acupuncture as a natural option is that contrary to massage (for instance), it tends to be utilized to treat the pain of any kind and in any region of the body because of the way that it is a totally comprehensive (entire body) way to deal with pain. While as a technique for relief from discomfort, massage is, in all respects, centered around disposing of muscle pain, acupuncture can be utilized to address any sort of pain, anyplace in your body.

This is one reason why acupuncture is ending up progressively broadly acknowledged by the customary western therapeutic clubs who are these days progressively liable to prescribe a mix of acupuncture and pain-relieving analgesics much of the time when pain should be managed.

For instance, this methodology is ending up progressively frequent with individuals who endure post-surgical pain. By giving a mix of acupuncture and pain-relieving analgesics, numerous specialists have discovered that they can totally free post-surgical patients of pain in a way in which analgesics all alone would have never been able to do while maintaining dosages at safe levels.

In contrast to numerous normal procedures for bringing alleviation from pain, acupuncture can be utilized to manage practically any sort of pain, a reality which is frequently overlooked or unreported.

For instance, numerous ladies report that acupuncture can be profoundly powerful for initiating labor and that a large number of the pains and worries of enduring pregnancy can likewise be soothed by acupuncture.

A few women endure back sciatica or back pains while pregnant in light of the extra weight, the pain of which acupuncture can altogether lessen. Numerous women likewise endure morning sickness and while acupuncture won't really make it go away entirely, it can give noteworthy assistance in decreasing the sickness levels that most ladies who are dealing with it feel.

It will do this by applying pressure on the Pericardium 6 needle acupuncture, which is inside the wrist. This is the system that has been demonstrated over and over to lessen all types of nausea, along with morning sickness.

As another option, you should consider utilizing a pressure point massage band to apply pressure on a similar acupuncture point as a method for lessening nausea brought about by morning sickness.

In the last trimester, numerous women endure pelvic support pain and as per Swedish studies, acupuncture can help with those pains as well.

The excellence of utilizing acupuncture to lessen the seriousness of the different pains related to pregnancy is that thusly, you decrease or expel the need to consume unnecessary medications. For certain ladies who have an intolerance to drugs, this is mandatory, however, regardless of whether you fall into this classification, it clearly bodes well to lessen your dependence on medications while a baby is being carried and during the birth procedure.

Another region of pain that can be managed exceptionally viably and productively with acupuncture is the alleviation of pain for cancer patients. Since cancer isn't just one illness (there are more than 300 various cancers) and furthermore, in light of the fact that chemotherapy treats the majority of the various types of cancer in an alternate manner, it is beyond the realm of imagination to expect that acupuncture is going to be useful for each situation.

As far as helping cancer patients get over their pain or nausea that is a typical side-effect of going through chemotherapy, acupuncture can be an important extra option in the pain management toolkit.

Would acupuncture be able to help cancer patients? Almost certainly, acupuncture can help under the watchful eye of professionals.

While it is reasonable to propose that despite everything, we don't generally comprehend why acupuncture is so successful as a treatment for pain, the staggering proof gathered for several millennia from medicinal specialists everywhere throughout the world is that acupuncture is a wonderfully compelling method for managing pain, practically regardless of how or why that pain happens.

In the event that you deal with pain, particularly, chronic pain that is probably not going to be managed by something that delivers brief and momentary help, acupuncture is unquestionably an alternative that you ought to consider.

Regardless of whether acupuncture all alone can give you the pain management you need or whether you have to utilize pain-relieving analgesics in the mix with this specific type of natural treatment, on the off chance that you can utilize acupuncture to diminish your pain, the number of analgesics you need is going to be also decreased.

Now and then, we may like to utilize natural medicines to manage pain, even if it is unfeasible to do as such every single time, especially when pain is especially extraordinary. For this situation, painkilling medications likely could be essential, yet in the event that they can be mixed with a natural arrangement like acupuncture to diminish the necessity of drugs, this decreases the danger and thusly the potential uncomfortable side-effects that you may deal with by consuming these medications.

Chapter 7: Hypnosis

Can Hypnosis help with pain?

While for most individuals from the general population, hypnosis is most ordinarily connected with humorously amusing stage demonstrations where individuals do obviously insane things or maybe with awful TV sitcoms, the perspective of the mental and medical community of what hypnosis is about is very different.

Since it was first developed by Franz Anton Mesmer in the 1700s, it has turned out to be progressively broadly acknowledged that utilizing hypnosis can manage or treat numerous apparently unsolvable issues, including the chronic pain management.

For quite a while, the western medical field tended to accept that finding an answer for an issue consistently involved not much more than temperature measurement and shot administration. Thus, the possibility that something as bizarre as hypnosis could have any certifiable influence in managing mental or medical issues was essentially a lot for individuals to accept.

Yet, the truth of the matter is that when deductively conducted by an expertly qualified hypnotherapist, hypnosis is a strikingly compelling procedure that can be connected to managing a tremendous scope of issues and challenges. For instance, hypnosis is frequently utilized as an exceptionally powerful method for persuading individuals to quit smoking while it is additionally used to treat the individuals who really need to quit drinking and other people who endure due to a comparably addictive or obsessive character.

Above all, throughout the last couple of decades years, hypnosis has been subject to the nonstop examination of numerous clinical preliminaries and in pretty much every circumstance, it has been demonstrated that hypnosis is a viable method for dealing with pain. Individuals experiencing pains related to cancerous growth, gallstones ,kidney stones, spinal pain and intrusive medicinal and dental treatments have all been subjected to hypnosis with striking success.

As per one noted specialist, Dr. David Spiegl M.D. of Stanford University, 'Changing your psychological state can change what's happening in your body', and the majority of the proof shows this is correct as far as managing chronic pain goes.

During the hypnosis, the subject is quieted into a condition of central fixation, inward focus in addition to laser-focused attention and all at the very same time as they are completely calm. Consequently, the subject in this hypnotic state can receive suggestions more successfully than they may in their cognizant state while they can likewise take advantage of unused mental forces to extend the limits of potential physical outcomes.

Throughout the years, numerous studies and papers have given convincing proof that hypnosis is exceptionally successful with regards to managing pain.

For example, in the April 29, 2000 version of 'The Lancet', there was a report contrasting the outcomes between patients under hypnosis and those under standard medical care who were experiencing intrusive medical procedures. The outcomes demonstrated that the patients who were hypnotized endured significantly less pain and uneasiness than the individuals who were utilizing typical painkillers.

Likewise, the medicinal procedure itself required impressively less effort to finish for the hypnotized patients, most likely in light of the fact that there was no need to continue controlling their pain and quieting their nervousness as there was with patients under an ordinary sedative.

What was also interesting was the way that post-surgery, the patients who had been hypnotized didn't even require half as much painkillers as the patients who just received ordinary anesthetic procedures.

This proves how hypnosis is utilized in mix with usual pain-relieving practices, despite the fact that there is no reason behind why it can't be utilized by itself in specific circumstances.

For example, Dr. Alexander Levitan, who is a therapeutic oncologist in Minnesota, reports that he has done numerous surgeries, including hysterectomies and tracheotomies, utilizing only hypnosis for relieving pain.

There are various theories about why hypnosis would work in such a circumstance, with some proposing that since hypnosis modifies what you expect as far as the upcoming pain is concerned, this influences how you experience that pain somewhat later. Then again, another theory proposes that hypnosis redirects the focus towards other things, which moves your main focus away from focusing on the pain.

There are numerous studies presently being done to find precisely why hypnosis is so successful in blocking pain, a large number of which are centered around physiological changes (the adjustments in your brain) that occur while you are under hypnosis.

From these studies, it appears to be likely that hypnosis fires up certain regions of the brain that are all about attention and focus. As a result, hypnosis empowers your mind to concentrate on something other than the pain. Along these lines, your brain is kept from bringing the pain that you were formerly enduring or were going to endure to present awareness.

Anyway, you realize that help with the pain is 100% conceivable by using hypnosis, the following question is, what will you do about it?

The first possibility is to get in touch with a hypnotherapist in your neighborhood who can help you by going through your issues, and afterward, hypnotizing you so that he could begin tending to your pain.

Finding an appropriate hypnotherapist

Before you go through with this, in any case, there are several things you ought to do. Right off the bat, you should talk with your doctor or medicinal professional, the individual who is currently tasked with keeping you healthy. Know that when you do as such, they may not be very happy with what you are considering doing, particularly as by looking for the assistance of a hypnotherapist, you are partially reducing their assistance and role.

Trust me, it is quite conceivable that your doctor will respond along these lines – in the event that they have been treating you from time to time, you presumably know them more than most, so you may have a proper expectation of how they are probably going to respond.

Be that as it may, the truth of the matter is, you are not there to request their suggestion or approval. What you have to know is whether exposing yourself to hypnosis represents any genuine dangers, such as the possibility that some current condition could be made worse because of the experience of hypnosis.

What you are searching for is the medical confirmation, so if your doctor does not endorse the possibility of you looking into hypnosis for any reasons other than those which are carefully medicinal, it is your choice whether you go through with it all.

Also (and assuming that you choose to proceed with attempting hypnotism), you have to discover a hypnotherapist who is fit for treating the issue that you will present to them. While most hypnotherapists will be able to manage more 'common' requests, for example, individuals who need to quit smoking and so on, few hypnotherapists will be able to deal with chronic pain without any reservation.

Thusly, you may need to contact a couple of properly qualified experts to see whether they can aid you. Visit them to see whether you can work with them. To put it plainly, you have to feel 100% relaxed with the hypnotist you are intending to work with since if that is absent, there is a component of stress or strain brought into the relationship which won't assist you with achieving the outcomes that you're searching for. The subsequent option is to learn self-hypnosis. Furthermore, if that sounds insane, get ready to reconsider!

Is Self-Hypnosis Possible?

Do you recall the last time you headed out to see a film at the cinema? In the event that you can and it was a famous movie, you were most likely not by any means the only individual in the room, yet only one of many energized individuals waiting patiently for the light to go down so the fun could start.

At the point when the house lights were shining, you were glancing around, very much aware of the rest of the audience, yet when the lights went down and the movie began, the movie was all you could think about.

In this circumstance, you have successfully changed your center of focus from this present reality of which we are, for the most part, mindful, to the movie and you have committed to it entirely. To remind of the cliché, this present reality has stopped to exist and the main world is that of the movie.

The idea of self-hypnosis isn't particularly different than this fundamental idea. It is tied in with moving and centering your focus, and the more effectively you can do as such, the simpler self-hypnosis tends to be.

Most reassuringly, it is ordinarily believed that the capacity to hypnotize yourself depends to an enormous degree on your willingness to do as such and your need to be in control of your pain. To put it plainly, most of the individuals who wish to control their pain through self-hypnosis figure out how to do as such by sheer resolution and their willpower.

Having some direction of how you can voluntarily control your attention is a valuable thing, especially toward the start, so counseling hypnotist who can assist you with developing your own capacities is probably going to pay off handsomely. Along these lines, you get the best possible direction from the starting point while being instructed by somebody who truly knows their stuff.

Then again, there are a lot of sites where you can get the hang of most that you would ever need to know about self-hypnosis, which has the upside of you learning self-hypnosis voluntarily and in the solace of your own home.

Perform a Google search for 'self-hypnosis techniques', in light of the fact that doing so will demonstrate to you how many self-hypnosis websites are out there.

While you will likely not be astounded to realize that most of these websites are selling products that have to do with self-hypnosis, plenty of them are stuffed with free ideas and material that are going to enable you to get the hang of all that you require for self-hypnosis.

When you do begin going a bit deeper with all the material, you may be be shocked to understand that the ideas or concepts behind self-hypnosis are not so bizarre or wacky as they may seem from the outset. Self-hypnosis is actually simply a twin stage procedure of unwinding as totally as could be expected under the circumstances and afterward concentrating on something that takes your thoughts off the pain that you are attempting to escape from.

The calm state that is usually associated with that of an individual in a self-hypnotized state is the unwinding that is felt by the individuals who meditate routinely.

What's more, as any individual who meditates each day will let you know, arriving at the degree of unwinding you require to accomplish your goals isn't something that occurs overnight.

To put it plainly, you have to figure out how to unwind as completely as could reasonably be expected, and after that, to continue with your unwinding strategies with the goal that you get increasingly effective and become progressively relaxed because of doing as such.

As insane it may sound, self-hypnosis is a successful method for managing pain in a natural manner. Simultaneously, in light of the fact that a basic piece of the self-hypnosis procedure is your capacity to loosen up more than you have ever managed previously, the general advantages for your wellbeing realized by the unavoidable decrease in strain and stress this causes are going to be a crucial part in the battle against pain.

There is one last alternative option that you may want to consider. I have said that a Google search will find numerous results that have to do with self-hypnosis items and services being sold on the net. A portion of these items, a significant number of which are CD or DVD introductions by expert hypnotherapists that are going to instruct you to try self-hypnosis at home may pose an opportunity that is worth the evaluation.

Chapter 8: Herbs for Pain Management

There are a lot of herbal remedies and herbs that are thought to have pain-relieving characteristics, in spite of the fact that it is commonly acknowledged that a great deal of these natural options are not as effective as the pharmaceutical options.

Thus, while the herbs and herbal medications suggested in this chapter of the book are going to deliver alleviation from certain aches and pains, they are probably not going to be powerful on the off chance that you are in outrageous, intense or extreme chronic pain. All these cures merit attempting on the off chance that you are in some pain and need to tackle the issue rapidly and naturally.

Willow bark

It doesn't come as a surprise to realize that willow bark is a viable herbal pain diminisher when you understand that the fundamental active compound in aspirin is a derivative of salicylic acid which is one of the three core components of the willow bark herb.

It was this association between the component in what is the world's most well known over-the-counter painkiller and the active ingredient in willow bark that initially proposed that it would be a fruitful natural painkiller. Sadly, in light of the fact that the speed of absorption of salicylic acid from willow bark is to some degree slower than the rate of absorption of its pharmaceutical cousin and since there exists such a difference in duration, the natural option isn't exactly as powerful as the chemical option.

Then again, there is some proof that a supported portion of willow bark over a week or so is going to begin to decrease back pain(a daily dose of 130 mg daily is prescribed), while different examinations recommend that an ordinary portion of willow bark can provide some alleviation to those enduring osteoporosis with no discernible side-effects.

In any case, this is a herb that ought to be avoided in the event that you have an aspirin hypersensitivity or endure gastric or peptic ulcers. Additionally, on the off chance that you are susceptible to gout, diabetes or have any type of liver or kidney ailment, you should not utilize willow bark.

Peppers

Peppers are a typical staple, all across the world these days, with different assortments of peppers, for example, jalapenos, chili, cayenne, paprika, pimento and more being accessible wherever throughout the whole year.

Peppers of this nature contain a substance called capsaicin and the spicier it is to eat, the greater amount of this substance it contains. As a result, capsaicin is the thing that gives it its warmth, and eating hot peppers can improve circulation, fortify the heart and sensory system, mitigate acid reflux and boost appetite too.

Nonetheless, it is capsaicin that makes peppers intriguing for somebody who experiences chronic pain since it is accepted that this specific substance can diminish the degrees of the protein that is thought to transfer pain signals from the nerve endings to your mind. In the event that the degree of this transporter protein, which is known as substance P can be decreased, it makes sense that your pain is going to likewise be diminished along these lines.

For instance, in clinical tests, creams containing short of one present capsaicin administered topically to a painful zone have appeared to facilitate the pain relief caused by cluster headaches and shingles just as post-mastectomy and post-amputation pain.

Ingested internally, capsaicin has been believed to help with overseeing different gastrointestinal issues as it reanimates the flow of digestive juices and there is some proof that the antibacterial characteristics of capsaicin can help diminish colds and diseases.

Boswellia

Boswellia tree that is noted for its fragrant resin, is likely a creation of one of the four primary sorts of Boswellia tree.

Boswellia sap or concentrate has for quite some time been a staple of Ayurveda, with some proof that it has anti-inflammatory properties and can be utilized as a natural treatment for asthma also.

In particular from a pain perspective, in a study of 30 patients experiencing osteoporosis of the knee, 1000 mg of Boswellia concentrate given over a time of about two months was proven to improve things significantly when contrasted with a placebo group.

Indeed, the improvement was in certain subjects noted to make the pain subside by as much as 90% with an improvement in utilization and mobility of the knee. Then again, no huge improvement was noted in the group utilizing the placebo.

While most specialists accept that more examinations should be done before the case for Boswellia as a characteristic painkiller is built up past all sensible uncertainty, the outcomes so far appear to be incredibly reassuring.

Cherry Fruits

The helpful impacts of the fruit of the sour cherry in people have not been examined to any extraordinary degree up until now, yet the way in which the fruit contains substances that restrain the development of inflammatory proteins in the very same manner as ibuprofen imply that there are some possibilities for pain relief.

Moreover, it is accepted that sour cherries contain antioxidant characteristics and that they might be powerful for inhibiting the development of colonic cancer and possibly different types of cancers.

Ginger

There is some proof that including doses of ginger in your dietary routine (normally or as a supplement) is going to balance the pain of osteoporosis and also, incorporating extra ginger in your dietary routine has no unfriendly side-effects either.

In tests, it was demonstrated that incorporating ginger concentrate in your day by day diet may lower pain levels from osteoporosis by a sensible amount while moving and standing and that general degree of rigidity brought about by the condition should diminish as well.

In any case, there is no proof that incorporating extra ginger in your eating regimen is going to diminish different types of pain too much or improve your general personal wellbeing if chronic pain is in question.

Curcumin

Curcumin is the core polyphenol compound that gives turmeric its flavor and yellow color. Turmeric is a part of the ginger family, for which we have just observed to have some painkilling characteristics.

From the perspective of herbal medication, curcumin has appeared to have amazing anti-inflammatory characteristics because it is accepted to contain a potent COX-2 inhibitor. Without a doubt, in one study, curcumin was demonstrated to be just as powerful as cortisone when it came to managing acute inflammation while it was half as potent as the medication for managing inflammation of the chronic kind.

Given these amazing anti-inflammatory characteristics, it is nothing unexpected that curcumin has appeared to help mitigate pain in conditions where inflammation is an indispensable factor in causing pain. Incorporated into this rundown of conditions where curcumin might most likely assist in lessening the pain are osteoporosis, rheumatoid arthritis, ulcerative colitis and fibromyalgia.

In spite of the fact that there are no clear side-effects from utilizing curcumin as a natural painkilling option, it isn't appropriate for individuals who have stomach ulcers, hyperacidity issues, or gallstones.

Conclusion of Natural Pain Management

As any individual who has ever endured intense or chronic pain is very much aware, when you are in pain, you have to take care of managing it. Also, while we can all presumably live with low-level pain regardless of whether it is consistent or not, it is common for your need to handle the pain to grow as it gets more annoying

There is no uncertainty at all that in the West, when pain strikes, the first idea or response is to rush off to the medication cabinet to see whether there is any pill to address the issue. All things considered, utilizing pain-relieving medications is easy and fast for the vast majority of us when we have a migraine or spinal pain and when there is a desire to dispose of it as effectively as possible.

Nonetheless, as you presently comprehend, pain-relieving medications can possibly cause uncomfortable reactions, some of which may be mellow; however, many are clearly not. As a result, each time you pop paracetamol or aspirin into your mouth, you are going out on a limb and while it is pretty easy to imagine it is a noteworthy risk, it is a risk that you are undertaking.

Instead of popping a pill when you're enduring a momentary pain, give herbs a try itemized in the last chapter or try something like going out for a long relaxing walk in the natural air. While this is anything but the innovative painkilling suggestion, a long walk is going to regularly clear a headache, while muscle pain can frequently be alleviated by getting those muscles in motion.

Obviously, on the off chance that you experience the ill effects of chronic pain, at that point, the option that you are looking for is increasingly a long term one and lasting.

That is why a portion of the natural pain management methodologies that you have read about in this book, for example, hypnosis or massage must merit considering. Despite the fact that it is reasonable that the idea of having long needles pushed into your body might be somewhat uncomfortable, you need to remind yourself of how much it would mean to score a win against the pain you are feeling.

Whatever sort of pain you experiencing the ill effects of, it is conceivable to bring that pain level down by applying the natural pain management techniques that you have read about in this book.

Thusly, you might diminish or even quit taking possibly destructive pain-relieving drugs, which in itself going to bring huge medical advantages and improvements in wellbeing and lifestyle.

It never truly bodes well to take possibly unsafe synthetic compounds when superbly legitimate natural choices exist. As you have read, there are many natural pain-relieving options that work, so it unmistakably bodes well to begin utilizing them as soon as possible.

I hope that you enjoyed reading through this book and that you have found it useful. If you want to share your thoughts on this book, you can do so by leaving a review on the Amazon page. Have a great rest of the day.

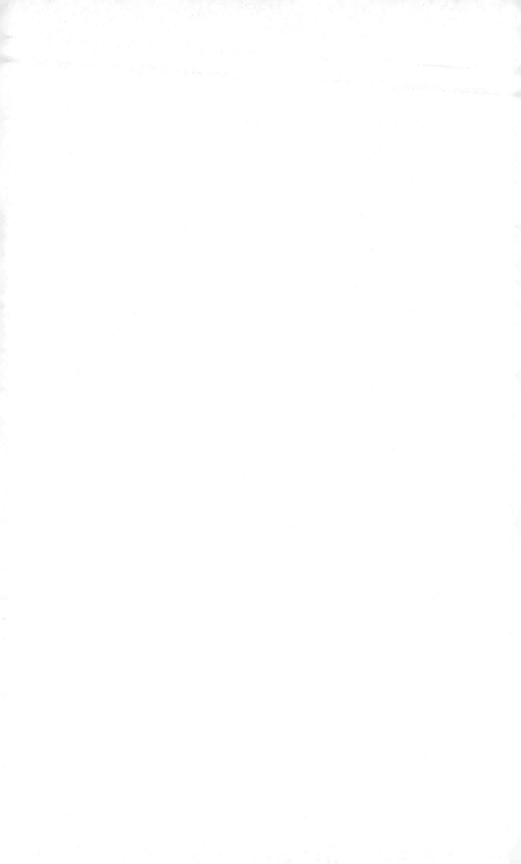

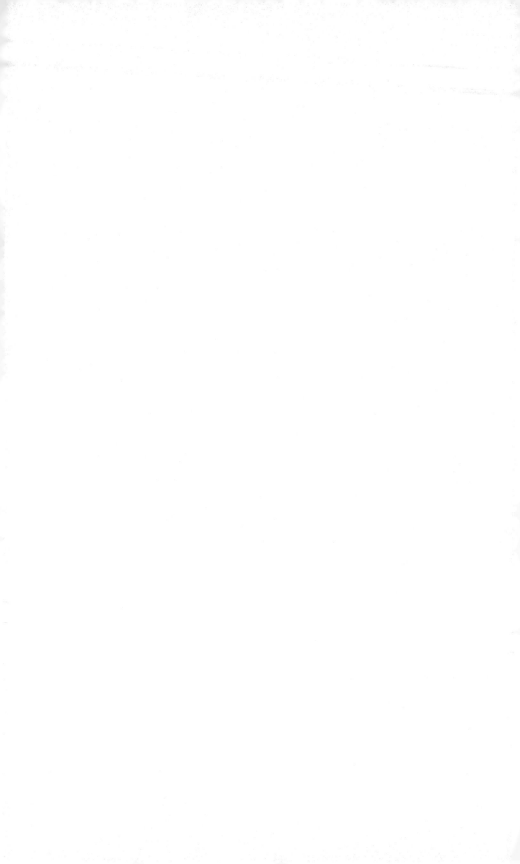

Made in the USA
Middletown, DE
21 August 2023

37125437R00136